INTEGRA...

A Balanced Account of the Data

Second Edition

Editor:
Steven Wirth, MD, MPH

Associate Editors:
Mary Farkas, MS, RD, MA
Peggy Miniclier, RN, FNP
Larry Reed, Pharm D
Sandra Wirth, RD

Consulting Editors:
Edzard Ernst, MD, PhD
William Jarvis, PhD

Cover Illustration:
Sue Ellen Parkinson

EDITOR: Steven Wirth, MD, MPH
ASSOCIATE EDITORS :
  Mary Farkas, MS, RD, MA
  Peggy Miniclier, FNP
  Larry Reed, Pharm D
  Sandra Wirth, RD
CONSULTING EDITORS:
  Edzard Ernst, MD, PhD, FRCP (Edin), Chair in Complementary Medicine,
Dept. Complementary Med., Univ. of Exeter, England. E-mail: E.Ernst@exeter.ac.uk
  William Jarvis, PhD, Executive Director, National Council For Reliable Health Information, Prof. Of Public Health and Preventive Medicine, Loma Linda University.
Cover Illustration: Sue Ellen Parkinson

© Copyright 1999, **Boitumelo Publishing Inc.**, (a Creative Logic company), 296 Toyon Rd., Ukiah, CA 95482. USA.
  ISBN 0-9661161-4-3. All rights reserved. **www.boitumelo.com**

Editor's Introduction

Patients have many questions regarding "alternative" therapies. In particular, they wish to know which of these therapies, if any, might be worth *integrating* into their health care. It was in response to such inquires that this book was conceived. The editors first looked for a suitable reference already available in print. Finding none, we set out to compose a table of herbs and nutrients to which we could quickly refer for answers.

Due to patient demand, our little reference work expanded to include other therapies not usually included by conventional practitioners of medicine. Throughout this process the editors have had continual testing of their reviews by patients. As the manuscript grew, the mission of this book remained to present to health professionals a practical, balanced account of the data regarding alternative therapies. Throughout, the emphasis is on practical, balanced analysis.

The first edition was well received, with the most frequent request being to increase the type size for improved readability. Not far behind my seasoned colleagues who suffer from presbyopia, I acquiesced to this concern, and so this edition is presented with normal type size. Beyond this, of course, we have reviewed some 200 recent reviews and original studies, and have included several new therapies.

Our approach is succint and "to the point"-- what you would expect to find in notes taken from a literature search done by practicing health professionals. As such, you will find very little prose here. What we trust you will find is a practical clinical reference. A list of useful web sites (page 133) will help the studious find even more detailed information. In addition, a bulletin board is available at the publisher's web site, www.boitumelo.com as an ongoing resource for readers. I hope you will also use that site to provide suggestions for the next edition.

The contributing editors are busy health professionals—ever at the "front lines" with the patients' needs and inquires. Ultimately, it is our patients who inspired this work. Beyond this, the quality of this project has been greatly enhanced by our consulting editors—Edzard Ernst, MD, PhD and William Jarvis, PhD. They bring honesty and keen academic knowledge to a field where such qualities can be difficult to find. For their assistance I am most grateful.

Steven Wirth, MD, MPH

February, 1999

TABLE OF CONTENTS:

Editor's Introduction	5
How to counsel patients	8
How should we evaluate unconventional therapies?	12
Key and Disclaimer	17
Critique of Therapies	20
Popular Diets	42
Systems approach to use of Complementary Therapies	52
Herbs and Selected Foods	81
Nutrient Table	112
Favorite Web Sites	133
References	135
Abbreviations used	163
Index	165

COUNSELING PATIENTS REGARDING UNCONVENTIONAL THERAPIES

Why bother to learn about such therapies?
If many of our patients are using unconventional or "alternative" therapies then we need to know how to counsel them. But *are* many of our patients doing so? Estimates of current use of "unconventional" therapies vary widely depending upon how inclusive one is when using this or similar terms. More inclusive surveys considered vitamins and exercise to be unconventional or "alternative" therapies. Other studies are more exclusive, perhaps not even including the use of chiropractic. It also matters how long a time period can have passed since the last use of such a therapy. Trying such a therapy once three years ago is different than daily use over an extended period. Not surprisingly, reported prevalence of the use of alternative therapies has varied widely, with figures ranging from 9% to about 60%. (602, 610, 611).

Even a 10% prevalence is significant, however. Many of our patients are using such therapies. Various forces have driven them to do so. For some, it is a sense of connection with a philosophy with which they feel comfortable (613), such as the notion that natural remedies are preferable to "high tech" ones. Many are simply looking for what ever may help them regain health, no matter whether it is classified as conventional or not. For others it is dissatisfaction with the rushed, impersonal care they have received from conventional sources. Peer influences, cost concerns, distrust of the medical profession and the belief in sensational anecdote lead others to the avant-garde. Furthermore, some of our patient's problems are not currently helped by conventional medicine. Few of us are so vain as to believe that we have all the diagnostic and treatment answers. How should we counsel our patients?

How should we respond to patients' inquires?
To borrow from an old proverb, we should do so with a marriage of kindness and truth. (603) Without kindness we will contribute to the feeling of isolation and depersonalization that drives patients away, at times, from highly effective treatments. Without truth we will do harm to our patients, our profession, and to ourselves. Through dishonesty patients are mislead and lose confidence in health care givers—a loss of confidence that may be a barrier to receiving future care. Devaluing truth also harms professionals intellectually as well as spiritually. (It can also ruin careers). If we are genuinely kind, our patients will feel more comfortable telling us what therapies they are using.

They will sense that we are genuinely interested in their well being. Hopefully this will foster a sort of teamwork between patient, health professional and the treatment offered.

Remember, two of the strongest predictors of a good outcome are the patient's sense that he or she can trust their doctor and the belief that their doctor is knowledgeable regarding their particular case.(604) To win trust we must tell the truth. With truth, including the admission of unknowns, the patient has the best chance to receive the most effective treatment. This responsibility to the truth includes the honesty to admit uncertainty and personal bias. Few physicians need reminding that this responsibility also means ever striving for more knowledge.

So a non-judgmental, supportive posture is clearly the way to address patients. Patients will also teach us a few things, and certainly as we listen, they will cause us to ponder new or forgotten treatments! At the same time, no matter what label is used, be it alternative, conventional, natural or integrative, there is no substitute for the *best* treatment. And the "best" treatment is preferably determined by peer reviewed research. In the absence of such research, or, more often, with incomplete data, one makes a judgment based on the available data, personal experience, and consultation with both patients and our professional colleagues. What we offer then is our educated opinion.

Checking the credentials of alternative practitioners:

If our patients do wish to consult a practitioner of an alternative modality, there are some further considerations. Foremost of these are: the likelihood of benefit from such a treatment, the qualifications of the alternative practitioner, and the determination of whom now is responsible for the outcome. For quality assurance and for liability reasons, it is important that his or her professional peers recognize the alternative practitioner as qualified in the area practiced. Such a health care provider should carry malpractice insurance and, if licensing exists for their profession, they should be licensed. A well-qualified professional would be expected to gladly volunteer documentation of such an inquiry by either the referring doctor or the patient.

Usually the responsible, experienced alternative practitioner would also welcome questions about what sort of cases he or she has most experience in handling. An advance request for feedback is also in order. If you feel certain alternative modalities may be worthwhile under certain circumstances, contact the professionals of those disciplines in your area and get to know them, if possible, before you refer. Also, check their credentials with their professional governing bodies, when possible.

Medico-legal concerns:
A jury may consider conventional health professionals who refer to alternative practitioners liable in the event of a poor outcome. In some cases conventional doctors are even considered more responsible, at least economically, than the alternative practitioner! To avoid being on the losing end of such a "heads I win, tails you lose" proposition, it is prudent to arrange timely return appointments with your patient in order to monitor progress. Do not abandon a therapy that has been proven to be effective in order to pursue an unproved one. Remember that you can refuse to be a part of such a mistake. When patients chose what you feel is excessively risky, tell them your opinion then document it. Do so with humility and respect, since in the future their choice might actually prove to be not so bad after all.

Counseling patients who self-treat:
Often patients are self-treating an illness and wish our opinion on their actions. It is hoped that this book will be highly practical in this setting. Patients acquainted with critical thinking in the academic sense may wish to study the relevant parts of this book as well. This is appropriate, provided they discuss it with their doctor before embarking on an unconventional course of action. Patients and health professionals alike will find the list of web sites on page 133 a handy resource for up to date information.

Sample questions to ask patients:
Beyond thinking through the above issues, it is useful to put into words a few questions that one can actually use during patient interviews. Feel free to create your own, but here are a few useful examples:

1) Are you considering the use of treatments not usually prescribed by medical doctors? (Such as herbs, vitamins, acupuncture, etc.)

2) Have you had any interesting experiences with alternative or unconventional treatments?

3) Have you had negative experiences with medical care?

4) If you do decide to use [acupuncture, homeopathy, etc.] do you plan to use conventional medicine at the same time?

5) Would you be willing to see me back in one or two [weeks, days, or relevant time interval] so we can see how things are going?

Specific questions to ask of an alternative health care provider include,

1. Tell me something about what you do.
2. What sort of cases do you like to see?
3. Are there some clinical problems that seem to respond particularly well to what you do?
4. Where did you train? How did you come to practice [acupuncture, homeopathy, the use of herbs, etc.]?
5. What sort of license or qualifications do you have in this field?
6. Are there risks to this treatment that we should be aware of?
7. Do you currently maintain some insurance in case of bad outcomes or malpractice claims?
8. Are there some patients of yours or professional colleagues that could provide recommendation for you?
9. Is there any particular religious or philosophic part of what you do about which patients may wish to know?

In summary, when counseling patients regarding unconventional therapies,

1) Be kind yet truthful
2) Use a non-judgmental approach
3) Consult academic sources, patients, and one's colleagues
4) Give your educated opinion regarding the therapy in question
5) Check the credentials of the alternative therapist to whom you may refer
6) Advise timely follow-up with the patient's primary care physician and/or relevant specialist

HOW SHOULD WE EVALUATE UNCONVENTIONAL THERAPIES?

The best medicine:
Respected authors have stated that there is no such thing as two separate kinds of medicine—one conventional and the other "alternative."(605) There is just the *best* medicine—medicine based on that which stands the objective tests of peer reviewed research. And then there is everything else. The face of medicine is always changing as such research goes forward. A decade ago peptic ulcer disease was largely believed by conventional medical doctors to be due to psychological stress. At first when evidence was presented that a bacterial infection by H. pylori was often causative, it was not believed. It took independent replication of the data by several other groups before we accepted the new discovery and changed the way we practice.

It may be that many such effective therapies and new ideas are "out there" in the world of alternative therapies. Some of these therapies belong to traditional healing arts that pre-date ours by thousands of years. And it may be that some of those alternative therapies are useless—or even harmful. How do we decide which are useful and which are not? The same way we decide any other proposed therapy—by the scientific method. Hypothesis is followed by a test of that hypothesis. Such a test must consider and control for possible sources of error and bias. Careful execution of the test or "experiment" is then followed by analysis and finally by conclusions. This whole process is then subject to criticism by peers and, where deemed of importance, attempts are made to replicate the findings by other, independent groups of scientists. Reviews then make sense of the bulky data.

We have studied and referenced many such original studies and reviews in this book. Throughout this book one will find letter grades which we assigned to the weight of evidence supporting most claims regarding a therapy, from "A" referring to excellent scientific support, to "D" being scanty. The criteria for assigning these grades are given in the key, page 18. Studies are also described in terms of "H" for human, "A" for animal and "L" for laboratory methods. (See p. 18 for key).

Ideally each assertion would be subject to a detailed meta-analysis, a rigorous method of review described a few paragraphs below. In the absence of huge amounts of time and money, the simpler review method noted above was used. Both analytic methods are the scientific foundation of this book. However, such methods may fall short in terms of addressing a social phenomenon wherein the use of alternative therapies grows rapidly fueled by popular opinion. Such popular acceptance of new (or old and forgotten) ideas is not peculiar to medical issues, and has been noted for centuries in health, economics, style and religion. (606)

An upside-down look at alternative medicine:

Many researchers believe that the ideal way to approach medical research is to begin with basic science, then work toward eventual applications and finally evaluate safety and efficacy in clinical trials. It is difficult, if not impossible, for such an approach to keep pace with popular use of alternative therapies. Some researchers, recognizing this, have taken a different approach to the whole problem. Instead of starting with basic science, this method starts with observation of what people are clinically using. It is therefore considered an "upside down" or "backwards" approach. The most notable of these is that of the Centre for Complementary Medicine at the Ludwig-Maximilians University in Munich. Their approach, under the direction of Dieter Melchart, is termed "scientific quality management." This basically means that they deal with the tremendous popular use of alternative therapies by combining clinical research with quality management. (608) Rather than start with detailed studies on the efficacy of a certain treatment, they began with a survey of what their population was doing. In other words, they first asked the question, "What is going on in the real world?" While screening for safety problems, they begin to ask, "Is there evidence for efficacy?" This question is considered from two points of view. First, do patients perceive the alternative treatment as effective? If so, then time and money may be spent to determine if the treatment actually does work on an experimental level. They then take a closer look at safety. The next question—Is it efficient? Is it cost-effective? Finally, can the therapy be improved?

In the United States, Eisenberg and colleagues performed the first step of the "scientific quality management" approach by conducting a survey to determine the prevalence of unconventional therapy use here. (602) This study was very inclusive in what it considered to be an "unconventional" therapy, and so prevalence figures were high. Still, it does serve as a landmark article which will help guide further research. Various studies have put the prevalence of alternative therapy use as anywhere from 9% when restrictive criteria are used, to nearly 60% when an inclusive posture was held. (610, 611) Beyond surveys and reviews, the progress of original research seems stalled due to lack of scientific and economic leadership. Hopefully this will be a temporary stall, however, and we look forward to well designed and performed studies on those unconventional therapies that are popular and/or promising in pilot studies.

Quantum theory, placebo effects and medical research.

Given the unusual philosophies that accompany some of the alternative therapies, it is not surprising that different ideas arise as to how to study them. In some cases, practitioners have objected to the whole notion of applying the scientific method to their "art," as in the resistance of anthroposophic medicine to usual research. A curious recent example of the mixture of science and philosophy has to do with quantum physics. Popularized recently by Andrew Weil in his book, Health and Healing, quantum theory is used to support the notion that our conscious mind can cause changes in matter which are otherwise unexplainable. In other words, miraculous healings are felt to be due to some inherent subatomic power of the conscious mind. Some promoters of alternative therapies go so far as to say that their therapies are not even subject to normal lines of scientific investigation because of the quantum theory. This would seem a non-sequeter from the work of the physicists who, struggling to explain how light behaves both like a wave and like a particle, developed the quantum theory to explain their observations. As Arnold Relman, editor-in-chief emeritus of the New England Journal of Medicine points out in a recent opinion essay, the leading physicists of our day consider the application of quantum theory to human consciousness to be unjustified. (605)

Another area of interest in scientific studies involving alternative therapies is the placebo effect. One's expectancy that one is being treated well has long known to have a positive effect—variously estimated to be significant from about one-third to one-half of the time in cases where psychological factors play a role, such as in asthma. Recent studies have looked as well at how the use of a placebo affects the results of controlled trials. (607) If a study subject receives a pill, not knowing whether it is active or placebo, they may be more likely to report improvement than a study subject who is given nothing. At least six published studies have evaluated possible biochemical mechanisms for placebo effects in pain control. These studies have used opiod antagonists and agonists to look for effects due to endorphin release when placebo is given. A recent review of these studies concluded that placebo analgesia does exist and that it occurs through the release of endorphins. (612) Respecting the effects of placebo, some controlled clinical trials are now including three study groups—those given active treatment, those given placebo, and those given nothing.

Meta-analysis:

Due to lack of funding, many published studies involving alternative therapies are small ones. Results from small or moderate studies may suggest trends but be non-conclusive. When results from similar studies are compared and the data combined, we have what is termed a "meta-analysis" or an "overview."

Combining data in this way can lead to conclusions that any of the smaller studies were too weak to support.

It is useful to note that such analyses are subject to errors due to dissimilar study design. Differing inclusion criteria are a problem as well. Further, it is well known that studies that show positive results are more likely to be published than those with negative findings. This is known as "positive publication bias." Better meta-analyses make a concerted effort to include unpublished studies in order to balance this effect.

Some health professionals view alternative therapies as inherently impossible to study in a scientific manner. How does one give a placebo acupuncture treatment, for example? Is there such a thing as a placebo massage? How does one prove or disprove the presence of the suspected "signal" left behind by the serial dilutions in homeopathy?

Research design.

Busy clinicians are most often confronted with research designed to prove the efficacy and safety of a prescription drug. That is where most of the money seems to be in medical research. Face it. How many drug company representatives have you met face to face in your office? Contrast this with the number of representatives visiting you in order to promote fresh fruits and vegetables in the diet, or to promote regular sleep and exercise!

The usual design of drug studies involves randomized, placebo controlled clinical trials. For those readers who heretofore have not bothered to figure out what that phrase means, briefly, randomized means that study and control subjects are chosen randomly; placebo controlled means, basically, that study subjects are given real treatment while control subjects are given fake treatment; and "control" means that attempt has been made to account for potential sources of error by building into the research design a means of separating out only the variable which one wishes to study. Often added to this is the notion of "double-blinded" which means that neither the researcher collecting the data nor the subject being studied knows, until afterwards, which individuals received placebo and which received the treatment in question. Such study design is very good, when properly conducted. However, it is not the only design worthy of inclusion in the term, "the scientific method." With the exception of the term "controlled" other features of study design are negotiable without obviating consistency with the scientific method.

Some modalities do lend themselves to double blind, randomized, placebo controlled clinical trials. Those that do not lend themselves to such tests require some ingenuity among those who design tests to evaluate them. Herbs can be tested in experiments similar to those used for pharmaceuticals. However, what would constitute a placebo for acupuncture?

How would you design a placebo to control for the effects of yoga? It takes a bit more creative research design to deal with such problems. But it can be done! It has been done in conventional medicine. For example, lifestyle studies such as smoking cessation, the benefits of exercise, and of eating fruits and vegetables were done using the scientific method but not using "placebo" cigarettes, "placebo exercise" or "placebo broccoli." A recent example in the field of alternative medicine was designed by a creative elementary student and was published in JAMA (548). Using the scientific method, Emily Rosa designed a test of the fundamental hypothesis of therapeutic touch—that a person's aura or presence could be detected through space. In a very cost effective experiment, the then 9 year old girl randomly placed therapeutic touch practitioners' hands over either another's hand or the table, hidden behind a blind. The practitioners could not predict when the other person was there, effectively demonstrating the failure of the previously taught belief of that particular healing art.

Acupuncture research has often used "sham" points or has been controlled in other ways, as with usual care not involving acupuncture. Some have proposed the use of laser acupuncture, which could give a non-penetrating, placebo laser or the penetrating one, as a meaningful design. Massage therapy studies have often used usual care as a control with the measurer of outcome being blind to which patients received massage and which did not. When patients are randomized to treatment vs. no-treatment, usual care or placebo, and when the person collecting the outcomes data is blinded as to which group the patient belongs, such studies are consistent with the scientific method. They are valuable studies and do help answer questions of efficacy.

Just because a study design is not obvious does not mean that we should ignore scientific inquiry. Such challenges just make the eventual discovery of truth that much sweeter.

HOW TO USE THIS BOOK:

This book is intended as a practical reference for health professionals, as well as for others who face questions about unconventional therapies. There are two basic ways these questions present—either as a question about the therapy itself, or as a question about a particular health problem. For this reason, the book has two main sections—the Critique of Therapies, starting on page 20 and the Systems Approach to the use of complementary therapies, starting on page 52. Most answers to questions raised by patients in this area of health, can be found in either of those two sections, plus the extensive table of herbs and selected foods (page 81), and the nutrient table (page 112). There is an extensive index (page 165) as well as a list of abbreviations (page 163) which are vital to efficient use of this reference. The Key and Disclaimer found on the next two pages are essential to proper use of this book.

Finally, the publisher's web site, www.boitumelo.com, with its bulletin board and e-mail capability, expand the usefulness of this book to its readers and provides opportunity to obtain more information from the editors.

KEY TO CRITICAL REVIEW OF LITERATURE:

(____:____; reference by number)

The letter to the right of the colon refers to the quality of the data found, as follows: "**A**" Refers to excellent supporting data. To earn an "**A**," the data was found to arise from: 1) scientific methods with appropriate use of statistics, 2) relevant design, 3) The data must come from consistently reproducible studies published in peer review journals, and 4) When possible, a randomized, placebo-controlled, double blind study design should be used. "**B**" refers to good data, with at least 3 of the 4 features of an "A" study. "**C**" refers to fair data, having at least 2 of the 4 features of an "A" study. "**D**" refers to currently poor or scanty data, having at least one of the 4 features of an "A" study.

The letter to the left of the colon refers to the type of study:

"H" for human,
"A" for animal, and
"L" for lab experiments.

REFERENCES (by number corresponding to list, p. 135) are given immediately after the above designation, or, in some cases, elsewhere in the vicinity—usually on the same line of text or same row in a table. The list of references, beginning on page 135, has citations sufficient to find the relevant documentation.

ABBREVIATIONS: please see page 163 for a list of abbreviations used.

DISCLAIMER:

REASON AND CAUTION: Most of the therapies mentioned in this book should be considered experimental, and insufficient data is present for health professionals to recommend many of them. Clinical judgment, along with the following considerations, should be used.

1) This handbook is intended to introduce the data that is available on a given topic or therapy. References are given for further study.

2) Recommending or referring for unorthodox therapies may carry undue risk to the patient while at the same time hold liability for the health professional.

3) Whether we like it or not, our patients are using many of these therapies. It is therefore prudent to educate ourselves about them, if for no other reason than to acquaint ourselves with the available data regarding these therapies. Contributing to such an acquaintance is the main goal of this book.

4) The vast need for more and better analysis of traditional and "alternative" therapies is humbling. Still, we must begin somewhere if we are to move toward intelligently answering our patients questions about what they may already be using.

5) Exhaustive efforts have been made to ensure the accuracy of this book. Still, inaccuracies cannot be completely excluded and no guarantee of accuracy can be made. The editors and publisher cannot be held liable for errors or omissions. Readers are advised to compare sources of information. The advantages of currently accepted norms of practice must always be considered.

6) Readers not wishing to be bound by the above statements may return their book for a full refund of purchase price.

CRITIQUE OF COMPLEMENTARY THERAPIES

GENERAL CONSIDERATIONS: Some of the more popular therapies used as integrative, complementary or alternative therapies are listed below in alphabetical order. For further critical analysis of any of these or other methods, the reader may wish to check the publisher's bulletin board on the World Wide Web at www.boitumelo.com. Also, readers may order specific up to date studies published by the National Council for Reliable Health Information— a non-profit organization that seeks to protect against health fraud and quackery. It may be useful to compare proponents information with that of the NCRHI. Their address and web site: 300 E. Pink Hill, Independence, MO 64057; http://www.ncahf.org.

While patients seek for and must be given the best available information, remember that there is an art to educating patients in such a way as to encourage their health, rather than to suggest that whatever they are doing is bound to fail, (the latter deemed the "nocebo effect") (407).

ACUPUNCTURE:
Description: Originating from oriental medicine (OM), it is often combined with OM's methods of diagnosis and other treatments such as herbs. The yin-yang principles are included which may advise herbs and lifestyle changes in addition to the acupuncture treatments. Traditionally, needles are placed in specific points on the body in order to up or down regulate energy ("Chi"). If more "chi" is needed at a specific point, heat (or burning a piece of herb on the blunt end of the needle—a practice called moxibustion) is added to the needle. The notion of "chi" is akin to that of "vitalism" which is present in many traditional healing practices. Practitioners may or may not believe that such a mysterious force actually exists. (See p. 33 for more discussion of vitalism).
Mechanism of action: In decreasing order from fair amount of scientific evidence to scanty, acupuncture may work by:
   1. stimulating endorphins (A:B;234)
   2. affecting the neuro-hypothalamic-pituitary axis (A:C;234)
   3. affecting the autonomic nervous system (A:D;234)

Effectiveness vs. specific illness: As one could imagine, it is difficult to reach consensus among scientists as to what constitutes adequate controls and good design in acupuncture studies. Our review of the data up to December of 1998 showed good evidence for efficacy of acupuncture in treating pain and nausea, with mixed or contradictory reviews in other areas.

Using our abbreviated format (see key on page 18) the data reviewed for acupuncture showed these effects:

Versus pain:
- effective Vs orthopedic pain (esp. low back pain)(H:B;234);
- effective in obstetrics vs. pain of labor and delivery, and to decrease time in labor (H:B; 528, 530);
- effective vs. painful diabetic neuropathy (H:C; 532);
- effective Vs fibromyalgia (H:C;271);
- effective Vs migraine (H:C;52);
- it has not proved effective vs. the pain of osteoarthritis (H:C; 535);

Other effects of acupuncture:
- **Vs medical problems:** anti-emetic (Vs nausea and vomiting) (H:B;234, 309); Vs asthma (esp. exercise-induced asthma)(H:C-;234); Vs insomnia (H:C;172); CVA rehabilitation (H:C;234); effective verses myocardial ischemia via decreased oxygen demand due in turn to decreased pressor response (A:B; 533); There is favorable data from a pilot study suggesting benefit in cases of urinary incontinence in spinal cord injury patients (H:D; 526). Acupuncture helped the clearance of skin infection in one animal study (A:C; 534); Specific effects for the treatment of obesity do not seem to be present (H:B; 411).
- **Vs psychiatric problems and addictions:** vs. depression (H:C; 536); Vs alcoholism is no different from placebo (H:B-;36); Vs other addictions (H:C-;234). Specific effects of acupuncture vs. various addictions, from alcohol and tobacco to "hard drugs" may be present, though we found contradictory reviews, perhaps underscoring the current difficulties in study design (H:C; 351, 433).

Many other uses have been described but are anecdotal, have poor design, have inadequate controls, (or we have not found them yet). In other cases the effects of acupuncture are not separated from other aspects of the total package of oriental medicine. Patient belief in this system, along with a polished tradition of practicing this art, may yield high success rates due to

"remembered wellness" even when specific therapeutic effects from the needles themselves cannot be explained. (see ref. 407).
Potential hazards of acupuncture: While usually safe when used by a licensed practitioner (see under "regulation" below), injury from the needles has been reported, including pneumothorax, damage to internal organs, bleeding, infection, (including viral hepatitis, AIDS, sepsis and endocarditis). Vasovagal reactions have also been reported. In a survey of 197 acupuncturists practicing in Norway, fainting during treatment was the most common adverse event, followed by a lesser incidence of increased pain (574). See reviews by Peterson (234), Norheim (574) and Ernst (412).
Regulation and referral: In the US there is prerequisite of 3 years in an approved school followed by successful completion of a nationally standardized "NCCA" exam. (Physicians already licensed need about 200 hours of training specific to acupuncture to qualify for the exam). For a list of qualified acupuncturists in your area call the American Association of Medical Acupuncture at 1-800-521-AAMA or visit their web site at www.medicalacupuncture.org.

ANTHROPOSOPHICAL MEDICINE:
Description: refers to the practice of medicine from a particular holistic view created by Rudolph Steiner (1861-1925). Steiner claimed to have received special revelations of the "spirit world" which led to over 300 published works in diverse disciplines including religion and science. Anthroposophy comes from anthropos "man" and "sophia" wisdom, referring to the wisdom that comes to believers when they can perceive both the spiritual as well as the material. It is taught at Waldorf Schools. In this worldview, philosophy and physiology are uniquely blended. For example, it teaches that humans have 12 senses, which correspond to the signs of the zodiac, and that actually the heart does not pump the blood. (580) Steiner was quite dogmatic in his teachings and rejected usual means of conducting scientific research. There are an estimated 1000 medical doctors who practice his brand of medicine in Europe, with another 50 to 100 doing so in the United States.
Evaluation of efficacy: not surprisingly given the apparent distaste for usual means of research, we could find little objective data evaluating this discipline. One review found that the methods basically amount to placebo effects and psychotherapy (575). A few reviews have looked for anti-cancer benefit from mistletoe extracts, one of this discipline's recommended therapies. Unfortunately, these studies found no benefit from its use. (577, 578). A few articles speak favorably of antrhoposophy's holistic approach to illness and disease (576, 579).

AROMA THERAPY:
Description: typically involves adding some aromatic oil to one's bath, inhaling its odor, or massaging it into the skin, for supposed health benefits. There is good evidence that recall of events learned in the presence of a distinct odor can be enhanced by the presence of the same odor at a later time. Other than this, there is little if any quality research into the various and often vague claims made by proponents of this modality. (599).

ART THERAPY:
Description: visual, or in some cases tactile, art participation and appreciation are used to treat illness.
Effectiveness Vs specific illnesses: Vs alcoholism (H:C-;98, 111); for adolescent psychiatric problems (H:C-;274, 312); for adult survivors of childhood abuse (H:C-;107); Vs dementia (palliative)(H:C;177, 285); Vs CA (palliative)(H:D;164); to develop empathy (H:C;229); Vs blindness (palliative use of tactile art)(H:D;94); Vs grief (H:C; 165, 260); rehabilitation (in general)(H:C-;242); Vs PTSD (and after abuse)(H:C-;107, 108); Vs schizophrenia (H:C-;302)

AYURVEDA: Description: meaning "knowledge of life" in Sanskrit, Ayurveda is Hindu traditional medicine, dating back to several hundred years B.C. Health is seen as a balance of mind, body and spirit, with diagnosis seeking to find the imbalance as well as the person's inherent constitution or body type. Treatment may involve "cleansing" (which may include purgatives and enemas) along with any of over a thousand herbs, and meditation.
Efficacy: Many of the herbs have been studied and found to be effective. Regular meditation is associated with a variety of health benefits including decreased BP and increased longevity. Scientific backing for these aspects varies from excellent, esp. for some of the herbs, to fair, such as with meditation (H:A to C; 340), to dubious for some of the bizarre traditional modalities, such as the use of milk enemas, goat feces, and other animal parts which we will not mention here,(581) and which hopefully have been abandoned by current practitioners!
Adverse effects: some remedies have had contamination problems, including by heavy metals.
Sources of more information: Ayurvedic Institute (505/291-9698). Compare with data from the NCAHF (http://www.ncahf.org)

CHELATION THERAPY:
Since atherosclerosis involves abnormal deposition of calcium deposits in arteries, chelation therapy attempts to demineralize such deposits as well as remove excessive amounts of heavy metals from the blood stream.

EDTA, deferoxamine and dexrazoxane are three of the more common agents used. The editors are aware of both positive testimonials and disastrous outcomes when attempts at chelation therapy resulted in delaying potentially life-saving usual care. This year a major review of literature published in this field over the past three decades concluded that "more controlled studies are required to determine the efficacy of chelation therapy in cardiovascular disease before it can be used broadly in the clinical setting." (H:B; 457). A recent review of its use in peripheral vascular disease concluded that chelation is no better than placebo. (H:B+; 597).

CHIROPRACTIC:
Description: Uses manipulation of the spine to treat back (or in some cases – neck) pain. Some chiropractors treat a variety of illnesses with manipulation as well as other modalities of their interest or training. Some traditional chiropractors believe their manipulations alter the "vital force" innate in living things. (See mind-body medicine).
Evidence of efficacy (or at least for increased patient satisfaction) is fairly good for the treatment of acute low back pain, (H:B; 365, 366, 589), fair for neck or shoulder pains, and the evidence drops off rapidly after that. In a recently published controlled trial involving 80 children, chiropractic was found to be ineffective in the treatment of asthma. (H:B; 590).
Potential hazards include vertebral artery dissection, excess x-ray use, some practitioner's expressed attitudes against immunization, and damage to nerves or even paralysis which is rare (H:B; 367, 368, 413, 414). Reported rate of vascular accidents is 1 to 4 per million manipulations. (413). Fractures have also occurred, esp. in patients with osteoporosis, in whom such manipulation is contraindicated. (413).
More information: for positive, promotional viewpoint see http://www.icacweb.com/ and for a critical view see http://www.chirobase.org/

ELECTROMAGNETIC RADIATION:
Description: refers to the use of electromagnetic radiation for healing, or, in some cases, to the adverse effects of such radiation. Depending upon type and dose, the effects can be either damaging or healing.
Positive effects: most data comes from photo (visible) radiation, (and heat and in the ultrasound used by conventional physical therapy), with some data for electrical and other sources.
    Bone healing: increased rate of fracture healing (H:B;10)
    vs. Multiple sclerosis: (picotesla doses)(H:D;255); visible light therapy (H:D;56)
    vs. Lupus: (UV A1 phototherapy)(H:C-;55)

vs. Circadian rhythm disturbances (such as shift work, insomnia and jet lag): properly timed bright light therapy, (and properly dark at other times)(H:B; 32, 72)
    vs. Seasonal affective disorder (H:A-;59) (Solar Lite 1-800-864-3883)
    vs. polio associated neuropathy—topically applied static magnetic fields of about 400 Gauss was effective in pain relief. (H:B—pilot study; 569).
    Vs. Psoriasis (H:A; usual care- moderate sun or therapeutic)

Negative effects (including some hazards of therapy):
    environmental excess: includes sun, radon, power lines, electrical appliances and transmitters: increased cancer incidence in children living close to power lines (H:C-;10); increased incidence of brain CA in electrical line workers (H:C;10); altered immune function (may be good or bad)(H:D;10)
    selected reported hazards of therapeutic radiation: besides the burns, gastrointestinal and reproductive effects of some forms of radiation, even phototherapy can have its problems, including burns, eye damage, skin aging or induction of skin cancer, and suppression of T-cell function which could adversely affect cancer or HIV patients, (1).

    Decreasing exposure to harmful radiation: shade and sunscreen offer protection in sunlight, (most sunscreens, except reflective ones like the opaque zinc preparations, form free radicals at the skin surface which raises some theoretical concerns over their use. Remember that radiation power drops very rapidly as distance from the source increases. Household sources of radiation include radon, electric can openers, electric shavers, hair dryers and vacuum cleaners. (10). Cell phones contribute some radiation of arguable relevance for the occasional user.

EXERCISE:
Benefits of regular exercise program including moderate, regular aerobic activity:
1. improved CNS function
2. increased endocrine capacity
3. increased energy capacity (i.e., more reserve energy)
4. increased efficiency of metabolic functions including oxygen transport and utilization, increased number of Na/K pumps, etc. (items 1-4 : H:A-C;310)
5. decreased risk of primary and secondary heart attacks (H:A;169)
6. decreased rate of age-related decline in immunity (H:C;270)

Benefits of exercise (continued):
7. improved immune function (with light to moderate endurance type exercises)(H:A;213, 214, 228)
8. to relieve stress (H:B;257)
9. therapeutic effect in rheumatoid arthritis
10. treating depression
11. treating peripheral vascular disease (H:B+; 593)
12. preventing and treating osteoporosis.

Potential adverse effects of exercise:
1. injuries (both acute and from chronic overuse)
2. heat or cold related
3. dehydration
4. exacerbation of asthma (least with swimming)
5. transient decreased immunity with prolonged vigorous endurance exercise (H:A;214, 215, 228)

Work site exercise has been evaluated by Shephard (269) who found the most cost effective programs were those which were built in to the normal day, especially walking or cycling to & from work.

HERBAL THERAPY: (see "Herbs and Selected Foods"- p. 81 ff., for evaluation of most commonly used herbs in this country.)
Description: The forerunner of modern medicine, herbs have been used traditionally for thousands of years to treat illness. It was from traditional uses that digitalis for heart failure, quinine for malaria, and caffeine for various uses was discovered. Herbs may be used for their specific physiologic effects, or in various traditional frameworks The popularity of herbs and supplements from them is growing much more rapidly than is the scientific basis for their use, partly in response to dissatisfaction with more "conventional" medical services. Studies of comparative strength and purity of the available commercial products have been few. The Herb Research Foundation should soon publish results of such a comparison of commercial ginseng products. The Los Angeles Times recently published an interesting comparison of St. John's wort products. They found that among ten brands sold, three had half or less of the potency listed on their label. One of the lowest potency, at 20% of the labeled amount, was from Sundown Herbals, a division of the nation's #1 dietary supplement distributor! (460).
Effectiveness Vs specific illnesses: With the above caveats taken to heart, there exists much data on the effects of many herbs. See "Herbs and Selected Foods," starting on page 25, for a summary and references. Or (for a reasonable fee) call the Herb Research Foundation @ (303) 449-2265 (web site: www.herbs.org) for information on a specific herb. In Chinese herbal medicine, herbs used are often little used in the USA, tend to be combined, and, at least in experienced hands, have been found effective, even in placebo controlled trials. (463).

Technical terms: an "infusion" refers to a tea. Typically one to two teaspoons of fresh or dried leaves or flowers are steeped in a cup of boiling water for 5 to 10 minutes. A "decoction" refers to a longer simmering in water, often of rough plant parts such as twigs, roots and seeds. A "tincture" takes advantage of a 20% to 80% ethanol in water mixture to yield the most possible active ingredients. Common tincture recipes call for herb:50% ethanol in water ratios of 1:4 to 1:8, with 12 or more hours of extraction time, and doses typically 2 to 5 ml at a time of the resulting solution. The best reference works detailing these preparation techniques for most herbs are those by Duke (406), Bartram (372), and Hoffman (373).

Adverse effects: Herbs and commercial supplements made from them vary widely in potency and are not always regulated. Despite popular opinion to the contrary, they can and do have harmful side effects (301, 413, 594). Such adverse effects have been reported due to allergic reactions, direct toxic effects, direct pharmacologic effects, mutagenic effects, drug interactions, contamination and by misidentifying the herb.(594). Tyler points out that misidentifying a plant can have fatal consequences. (301, p. Xii-Xiii).

HOMEOPATHY:

Description: Conventional western medicine often attempts to counter-act the agent or effects of a disease—thus the term "allopathy" meaning "opposite to disease." Homeopathy attempts to prod the body to health by presenting infinitesimal doses of substances, which, if given in larger doses, would cause symptoms similar to the disease—hence the term, "homeopathy" meaning, "similar to disease." The practitioner of homeopathy takes a very detailed history from the patient, trying to best match their particular set of symptoms with a specific "remedy." Though temporary worsening referred to as an "aggravation" may occur, healing is supposed to occur with the most serious problems showing improvement first. (142)

Homeopathy originated from the lifework of Samuel Christian Hahnemann (d. 1843), who also advocated exercise, proper hygiene and religious aspects of healing. (115)

Homeopathy remains popular in Europe, with up to 40% of conventional physicians either prescribing it or referring patients to someone who prescribes it. In the USA, the figure is closer to 1 to 2 % but is rising rapidly. (142)

Possible mechanism of action: remains largely speculative. Even proponents suggest the placebo effect may be responsible, others point out that there are multiple placebo-controlled, double blind trials that have published positive effects. (142). Benson notes that placebo, or "remembered wellness" works up to 60 to 90% of the time (407). Placebos are most likely to work when either subjective measures of outcome are used or in those illnesses in which the mind-body interactions play a large role, such as in asthma, hypertension and peptic ulcers (301, 407). See also "mind-body" medicine, p. 32 to 34.

At 12C dilution, the probability of finding a single molecule of the original, is essentially zero. (142, p. 32-33). Classic homeopathy holds that the more potent remedies are actually the more dilute ones! Ways the solutions may keep some sort of "signal" of the original substance, have been summarized by Jonas (142), with clathrates seeming the most favored theory at present. Clathrates are unique patterns of water—analogous to snowflakes. The actual experimental data supporting these mechanisms is very scanty and has not been reproducible.

Since history taking in homeopathy is detailed, visits are usually much longer than primary care visits to an allopath. The remedies are prescribed in such a way that one gets a very personalized prescription—a "close fit" for the symptom complex. Does this time for attentive interaction, together with the placebo effect and possible positive publication bias account for the reported benefits of homeopathy? With the relative absence of ceremony or ritual in Western medicine, does homeopathy find success by filling that void with a system of situation-specific symbols? Or are there really signals left behind in those dilute solutions, which affect physiology in such a way as to heal patients? Could part of the apparent success be the selection of diseases with immune or self-limited courses? Is there an interaction between the remedy and lifestyle changes advocated, (as with Hahneman's hygiene and exercise advise)?

Technical aspects: "X" refers to a 10 to 1 dilution. "C" refers to a 100 to 1 dilution, and "M" refers to a 1000 to 1 dilution. The number in front of the "X" or "C" refers to the number of serial dilutions. For convenience, the resulting solutions are usually poured over an absorbent material, such as lactose, to make the pills, which are then bottled and dispensed to patients or sold, in stores or through catalogues. A variety of things are traditionally believed to neutralize the beneficial effect of homeopathic meds: touching the medicine with one's skin before swallowing, coffee, contact with organic solvents, dental work, electric blankets, etc. (142).

Reported side effects: (81, 142): temporary worsening of symptoms, failure to use conventional therapy known to be effective and available, incorrect diagnosis, improperly made homeopathic preparations. Temporary worsening is often considered a normal process of healing, termed a "healing crisis." Such a belief in the face of serious illness can be life threatening. Homeopathy may represent a barrier to receiving immunizations or effective conventional care. (H:B; 81) There is at least one published report of a "homeopathic" drug that was found to contain pharmacologic amounts of corticosteroid (341). Conventional physicians who prescribe or refer for its use may face increased liability or board disciplinary action, (few states currently recognize homeopathy as a valid healing practice). Though apparently unusual, a fatal case involving homeopathy and malpractice has been reported (247). Perhaps the remedies themselves, (when unadulterated with actual drugs) are safe, but the judgment of those who prescribe homeopathy can be dangerous.

Published peer reviews and randomized controlled trials: (to look for efficacy): Klaus Linde and colleagues published the results of an extensive meta-analysis in September of 1997 to answer the question, "Are the clinical effects of homeopathy placebo effects?" (458). Their analysis argues that the clinical effects are not entirely due to placebo. However, they also found that there is insufficient evidence to say that homeopathy is clearly effective for any specific clinical problem. Such a conclusion lends itself to lively discussion. (459) Not surprisingly, selected excerpts of their conclusions have been quoted both by proponents of homeopathy and by skeptics. An earlier, well done review of research up to 1991 has been published by Kleijnen (150) which suggests positive, but inconclusive results—more, better studies needed. Since then, positive results for allergic asthma have been presented by Reilly (H:B; 342). Jacobs published positive results Vs childhood acute diarrhea (H:C;140). Soon thereafter, the same journal (Pediatrics) published a detailed analysis of Jacobs' paper, which questioned the positive conclusions of the first paper. (592). Michael Weiser published positive results vs. vertigo (H:C; 464). The following RCT's done since Kleijnen's review have also been published, but have yielded negative results: Vs rheumatoid arthritis (7); Vs plantar warts (343); Vs trauma (9); Vs upper respiratory infections (60); vs. Post operative dental complications and pain (173); and vs. Mosquito bites (127).

Sources of information: for a critics view, write to the National Council for Reliable Health Information, 300 E. Pink Hill Road, Independence, MO 64057, or contact their web site: www.ncahf.org. A summary of criticism of homeopathy was, admirably, published in the British Homeopathic Journal in January of 1998. The article, written by Edzard Ernst, should be required reading for both critics and proponents of this healing modality. (595). Detailed, favorable information, books, elaborate diagnostic and prescription computer software and even the remedies themselves are available from the Homeopathic Education Service, (1-510-649-0294; web site: http://www.homeopathic.com).

LIFESTYLE:

Healthy habits: Habits associated with longevity—no smoking, moderate use of alcohol, eat breakfast, no snacks, sleep seven to eight hours every night, exercise regularly and maintain proper weight. Those with all seven habits had a standardized mortality ratio of 0.6 compared to 1 for those with 4 to 5 habits and 1.6 for those with 0 to 3 habits. (H:B;78).

A 1993 review by McGinnis identified the non-genetic factors that are responsible for deaths in the United States (187). With his colleagues, he was able to provide estimates of the number of deaths that result per year in the USA due to preventable causes. These factors add up to about 50% of all deaths, the rest apparently attributable to genetic or unknown causes.

Non-genetic causes of death in the USA:

Cause	deaths/year	% of Total
Tobacco	400,000	19
Diet/sedentary	300,000	14
Alcohol	100,000	5
Microbial agents	90,000	4
Toxic agents	60,000	3
Firearms	35,000	2
Sexual behavior	30,000	1
Motor vehicles	25,000	1
Illicit drug use	20,000	<1
Total	1,060,000	50

Regular siesta is associated with lower average BP (H:B, 415), decreased risk for coronary artery disease (H:C, 415, 417) and, by inference, with less motor vehicle accident deaths (H:C, 416).

Does the practice of healthy habits lead to a prolonged, miserable old age? Vita and colleagues at Stanford recently answered this question in a lifestyle study of 1,741 Stanford alumni (582). Surveying their health habits, then following them for 32 years, they found that onset of disability was postponed by five years in the group practicing more healthy habits. Those with healthy habits tended to live longer and their disabilities were postponed and compressed into fewer years prior to death.

Traditional Chinese medicine includes a balance of lifestyle habits. Though seldom given credit for it, (probably because we do not emphasize it enough), conventional medicine includes advice in healthy habits which are supported by scientific data, such as proper nutrition, hygiene, regular exercise, avoidance of smoking, etc.

Religious groups studied for the health benefits of their recommended lifestyles have suggested benefits, (in some cases of varying habits)—such as in Orthodox Jews, Mormons and Seventh-day Adventists (SDA). These groups advocate no smoking, moderate or no use of alcohol, and offer educational, social and spiritual development. Even with well-defined study groups it can be difficult to sort out which variables are responsible for the apparent health benefits. Among SDA's, a vegetarian diet is recommended but not required. As such, in California about half of SDA's are vegetarian and half are not. When compared, the vegetarian SDA's have less heart disease and less cancer of most types, (except prostatic and uterine), and have a lower mortality rate. (H:B; 90, 91, 192). The protective effect of a vegetarian diet on cancer incidence was actually most closely associated with high intakes of plant-based foods, rather than the absence of meat in the diet (H:B; 192).

Studies on the health effects of faith and other aspects of spirituality are covered briefly on p. 74 to 79. See also "Mind-Body" medicine—p. 32.

MAGNETS: see electromagnetic radiation, p. 24.

MARTIAL ARTS: Includes qi-gong (essentially tai chi chuan), which is a discipline of slow moving mimicked battles emphasizing balance and flexibility. Observed benefits may include: effective vs. pregnancy induced hypertension (H:C, 477); maintenance of physical fitness, the prevention of falls, especially in the elderly (H:B, 471-6); treatment of stress and anxiety (H:C; 474).

MASSAGE THERAPY:
   Description: Falling under the more broad classification of "manual healing," massage therapy involves manual soft tissue manipulation. Swedish massage emphasizes long strokes, friction and kneading. Deep muscle and connective tissue massage aims for the deeper layers of tendon, muscle and fascia. These two techniques have the best scientific data supporting their effects. Esalen appears to be an effective stress relieving technique that emphasizes mind-body aspects. Less supporting data was found for techniques which apply mainly mind-body or "Chinese meridian" concepts, such as acupressure, Shiatsu massage and reflexology.
   Health benefits: Decreased lymphedema, (eg., post surgery, esp. after mastectomy) (H:A;344, 345, 346); versus anxiety and perceived stress (H:A;347); and for chronic pain management (H:A;348). Good to fair evidence exists for using massage in treatment of many health problems, with excellent data for neonatal applications, musculo-skeletal conditions, and conditions in which alleviation of anxiety is important (349, 350).
   Potential hazards of massage: Adverse effects can occur through mechanical means—such as the dislodging of clots in vessels to form emboli, or the spread of infection, or by physiologic effects, such as the worsening of CHF with massage which causes more

increased lymph and venous return to the heart, or the lowering of blood glucose, (351).

Confirmation of the certification of massage therapists and more information can be obtained from the National Certification Board for Therapeutic Massage and Bodywork. Phone: 1-800-296-0664; Web: http://www.ncbtmb.com.

Referral information: (the state chairpersons' numbers are subject to change). International- Contact AMTA National Office, 820 Davis St., Ste 100, Evanston, IL 60201-4444 (PH: 847-864-0123). State chapters of AMTA for referral:

AL- 205-349-3910	AK: 907-337-4478	AZ: 520-887-8819	AR: 501-524-9206
CA: 510-939-2682	CA res. Only 800-696-2682	CO: 719-594-0232	CT: 203-874-2476
DC: 202-332-0887	DE: 302-994-9089	FL: 850-445-0395	GA: 770-456-0009
HI: 808-988-1088	ID: 208-524-1696	IL: 708-275-1036	IN: 317-429-5516
IA: 319-377-7307	KS: 316-640-4241	KY: 502-776-0790	LA: 318-477-5770
ME: 207-729-9376	MD: 410-298-0704	MA: 508-534-8888	MI: 810-960-0959
MN: 612-696-1176	MS: 601-484-5710	MO: 573-964-0045	MT: 406-256-5694
NE: 308-381-7750	NV: 702-786-9499	NH: 603-668-4613	NJ: 732-748-0900
NM: 505-392-6744	NY: 212-925-7824	NC: 919-481-4141	ND: 701-872-4895
OH: 614-792-8255	OH res. Only 800-281-6548	OK: 405-943-6281	OR: 503-245-6810
PA: 610-838-1826	RI: 401-732-1140	SC: 864-599-0037	SD: 605-348-6942
TN: 423-886-6743	TX: 817-870-1340	UT: 801-393-9604	VT: 802-365-9414
VA: 703-519-5612	VI: 809-778-8018	WA: 206-528-6829	WV: 304-522-4781
WI: 608-231-9122	WI res. Only 800-482-2682	WY: 307-635-0839	

MIND-BODY EFFECTS AND THERAPIES:

Contrary to some of their critics' claims, practitioners of standard medical care are aware of mind-body effects and are not ideologically dedicated to the Cartesian notion that mind and body are separate, and that they do not affect each other. In fact, at times modern medicine has been slow to recognize "physical" causes of disease, therein over-stating the import of emotional factors. For years peptic ulcer disease was thought predominantly due to psychological factors. The discovery of Helicobacter pylori as causative was met with considerable resistance at first!

Many self-proclaimed "mind-body" systems are not holistic as they claim, but are dualistic (see below). Dualistic systems are generally "mind-centered," and assign the body a lesser role in health. Ayurveda teaches that the material world is an illusion and the unseen, ethereal world is reality. Christian Science teaches that disease and death do not exist. They are mental aberrations that only exist in corrupted human thinking. Many "alternative" health disciplines and their practitioners believe in a metaphysical life force that can be controlled to a great degree by the mind. The premise that such a "life force" imbues all organic molecules was a popular belief used to explain how homeopathy supposedly worked. It was believed that organic molecules could not be formed in the lab because man does not have the power to imbue that "life force" or "vitalism." Similar beliefs are still held by some practitioners of Ayurveda, chiropractic, acupuncture and therapeutic touch. However, this "vitalism" argument was discredited when Friedrich Wohler synthesized urea in the lab in 1828. Some Homeopaths, traditional chiropractors, Naturopaths, Ayurvedic physicians and acupuncturists believe that they are affecting such forces by their treatments while others, acknowledging this tradition, do not believe such forces are involved.

Holism (Wholism) versus Dualism: An exegetical examination of the concepts of body and soul (or spirit) in the Bible revealed that man was viewed as a whole being, not a dualistic being. The dualistic body-soul concept was a product of Eastern and Grecian philosophy. In the Old Testament, no Hebrew word can be translated as "body." The Hebrew word that is translated as "soul" in English refers to the psycho-physical totality of human beings. In the Old Testament, humans do not have souls, they are souls. In the New Testament the word soma is translated "body," but in Paul's usage it meant "personality"—the whole person. (583) It is dualism that separates existence into material (temporal, corrupt) bodies and ethereal (eternal, incorrupt) spirits.

Dualists can believe in such notions as so-called "astral projection" in which the consciousness can leave the body and travel outside of the "time and space" continuum (also known as "out-of-body" experiences). Some dualists believe that a drug-induced "out-of-body" hallucination is an ennobling experience to be sought after. Holists hold that humans are unitary creatures; that the mind is the process of the functioning human brain; and, that any thing that diminishes brain functioning reduces humanness—the ability to think and to do. Holists put a high value on physical health because it is inseparable from spiritual, mental, and physical health. There is no important difference between the way a holistic (wholistic) theologian or a neurophysiologist would interpret an "out-of-body" experience. Both would see it as the result of an upset in brain chemistry and distorted sensory perception. Much of what claims to be "holistic" is simply mind-centered instead of body-centered health care. In fact, ayurvedic apostle Deepak Chopra belittles material existence as being an illusion and venerates the ethereal as the true reality. Further, when pseudo-holists refer to the "mind," they mean the metaphysical "spirit."

"**Spirit**": There are many ways to use the term spirit in English. As emotion: a spirit of patriotism; as attitude: a spirit of worship; as spunk: an athlete with great spirit; as vigor: a spirited horse; as courage: a fighting spirit; as a personality trait: a virtuous spirit; as alcoholic beverages: distilled spirits; as ghost: a disembodied spirit; as philosophical values: spiritual aspects of life; as breath: inspire means to "take a deep breath." Some use spirit to refer to the breath of life God blew into Adam's nostrils to transform him from clay to "a living soul," and/or to refer to an attitude as in a spirit of worship. Some use spiritual to refer to philosophical values and a virtuous character. Those who hold a holistic view of humankind do not use spirit or spiritual to imply the existence of a ghost (soul, astral body, separate consciousness or existence) that is separate from material existence. There is no conflict between the holistic and scientific views of human existence.

Below are some **researched effects of the mind on the body:**
Immune function is improved with emotional well being, including perceived good social support. Immune function is impaired with unhealthy expression or inhibition of emotion or perceived poor social support. (H:A;352-357). The quality or disruption of one's marriage is included in these effects. (H:B;358). Besides infections, allergies are affected by one's moods (H:B;359).
Specific infections studied and found to occur more frequently or be worse in those under various kinds of stress:
1. the common cold (H:B;352)
2. herpes (H:B;356)
3. bacterial infection (A:B;152)
4. viral infections in general (A:B;152)

Mechanisms demonstrated for how the mind affects the body include via the hypothalamic-pituitary route, the autonomic nervous system, and via changes in neutrophil adherence (H:C; 116 and other studies)
Specific therapies:
1. **Biofeedback** has been successfully used to treat insomnia, anxiety and phobias, excessive muscle tension, GI motility disorders (H:C;86), TMJ problems (H:C;66, 326), athletic performance, and sexual dysfunction.
2. **Humor** when appropriately used decreases stress and improves both healing and coping. (H:B to C;180, 256, 324)

3. **Hypnotherapy** works in a fair number of individuals with some illnesses including acute pain (H:C-;137); irritable bowel syndrome (H:B-;89); relapsing duodenal ulcer (H:C;89); trichotillomania (H:C-;51); sexual dysfunction (H:C-;13); Urinary incontinence (H:D;13); chronic pelvic pain (H:C-;13); pain of childbirth (H:C-;13).
4. **Relaxation training** helps those with chronic pain (H:A;218) and alleviates insomnia (H:B-;218). To order relaxation tapes contact the Mind/Body Medical Institute at 617/632-9525 (USA).
5. **Meditation** (H:A; 407, 409)
6. **Belief**—in the idea that healing will occur, or that power(s) greater than ourselves are acting on our behalf. (H:A; 407).
7. **Helping others** without expectation of reward, (altruism). (H:B; 407).
8. Others such as art, music, and spirituality are mentioned under their own heading. Others, and to some degree all, therapies have some degree of mind-body interaction.

MUSIC THERAPY:
Description: Music, often self-selected, is used in a complementary manner to help in the treatment of illness or alleviate anxiety before, during or after surgical or diagnostic procedures.
Efficacy in specific settings: vs. Alzheimer's (palliative)(H:C-;3); to increase athlete's ability to relax at appropriate times and thus improve performance (H:C;26); Vs anxiety in medical or surgical settings, such as during chemotherapy, during flexible sigmoidoscopy, in intubated or ICU patients, (H:B to C;49, 251, 360); Vs aphasia (melodic intonation therapy)(H:C;19); Vs autism (palliative)(H:C;320); Vs dementia (specifically Vs repetitive disruptive vocalizations)(H:C-;43); Vs other aspects of dementia (H:C;243); Vs insomnia (listen before going to bed)(H:C-;199); Vs pain (palliative)(H:B-;219); in pediatrics (esp. to decrease newborn agitation and autonomic lability in the NICU)(H:C;40, 126, 144); other applications in pediatrics (palliative/adjunct)(H:B to C;151); Vs schizophrenia (palliative)(H:C-;139); stroke rehabilitation (H:B-;240); surgery settings, esp. peri-operative anxiety (H:C;109, 240, 321).

NATURAL HYGIENE:
Natural hygiene is one of several health movements that, to our understanding, arouse in reaction to the use of dangerous, ineffective and harsh treatments used by medical doctors in the USA in the 1700's and 1800's. Emphasis is placed on a healthy lifestyle and the use of such modalities as fasting, rest, nutrition and exercise to restore health. Many of the practices recommended make sense from a physiologic and hygienic viewpoint. Some

of these are well supported by research. However, some ideas taught do not have such support, such as the teaching to avoid certain food combinations at any given meal. For a recent review, see Shelton (267). As with many "alternative therapies," some generally sound advice can be harmful if it leads patients to neglect conventional treatment or preventive measures that have been proven to be effective. Natural Hygiene has been popularized by three recent best-selling books: Maizel's The Beverly Hills Diet, Diamond's Fit For Life and Robbins, Unlimited Power. (Contact the NCAHF for a critic's viewpoint).

NATUROPATHY:

Naturopathy is in two states at least, an officially recognized health profession, and basically consists of diagnosis and treatment without the use of prescription drugs. They may practice alone or in association with a conventional physician. In some cases they may rely on other (conventional) practitioners for diagnosis. A few, otherwise fairly conventional medical groups, have included a naturopath in their offices and consider their services as being part of the total services they provide to their patients.

Unfortunately, there are still persons promoting themselves as Naturopaths who have training from a variety of unaccredited programs, including correspondence schools. Apparently the American Association of Naturopathic Physicians is more particular in whom it recognizes professionally. Members are made up primarily of graduates of Bastyr University (Seattle) and the National College of Naturopathic Medicine (Portland, Oregon). Graduates of these two schools largely control the Council on Naturopathic Medical Education, an accrediting agency recognized by the U.S. Office of education. Under their auspices, at least, granting of the Naturopathic Doctor degree, "ND" requires a four year program which combines didactic and practical, supervised experience. Some MD's have become ND's, a process that can be accomplished in two years. Modalities taught and variously used by any particular ND, include the use of herbs, nutrition, homeopathy, acupuncture, physical therapy techniques, and mind-body techniques. Practitioners may or may not use all of these modalities. The extent to which they respect conventional medical and scientific approaches may also vary.

Naturopathy's attention to prevention by lifestyle, self-care, and conservative healing methods appears to be much like the general beliefs of Preventive Medicine, an established specialty of standard medicine. Hopefully we will be seeing more respect for this area of commonality rather than the all too familiar jabs at the "allopathic" straw man, which is typical of anti-science practices. Historical opposition to proven preventive practices such as immunization, fluoridation and pasteurization are reminders of some Naturopath's antiscience ideology. At the same time, many

Naturopaths promote Vitalism (Vis Medicatrix Naturae), resulting in a tendency to overstate the body's self-healing power, and they promote the beneficence of "natural" remedies (e.g., whole herbs alleged to be superior to drugs extracted from them).

Naturopaths have claimed to be the inheritors of the Hippocratic tradition because of their belief in Vis Medicatrix Naturea.(586) One could argue, however, that this belief in a mysterious "life force" reveals that these Naturopaths do not understand the most important point of Hippocrates' premise that the healing power of nature was not a mysterious force. "Naturopathy" is an Anglicized version of the term "physician" coined by Hippocrates who used the root word physikos—the Greek word for "nature"—to denote that every practitioner of medicine was to be skilled in nature and must strive to know what man is in relation to food, drink, occupation and which effect each of these has upon the other.(584) By this Hippocrates meant to displace the idea that disease and healing were dispensed by the gods (ie, supernatural forces).(585) It would appear vain for this discipline to claim a particular link to Hippocrates.

Conclusion: Many of the nutritional, exercise and stress management principles taught are useful and well supported by research. Unfortunately some of the more popular naturopaths use a mixture of valid and invalid handling of scientific data which misleads. Some naturopaths may cause harm by acting as a barrier to the use of proven therapies or vaccines. Further, some have held to the belief that when a patient is appearing more ill – a "healing crisis" is taking place, (similar to homeopaths' belief). Such a notion can be dangerous when it results in the delay of effective treatment in the face of serious pathology. On the other hand, there may be a trend toward a more integrated approach with "allopathic" medicine, and we are aware of at least one school of naturopathy which participates in outcomes research, (The National College of Naturopathic Medicine, located in Portland Oregon).

NUTRITIONAL THERAPIES:
See also under "Systems" for critiqued list of nutritional approaches to specific health problems, (p. 52), and under "Nutrition Table" for summary by vitamin, mineral, or specific nutrient, (p. 112).

DASH DIET (Dietary Approaches to Stopping Hypertension): The DASH study, published in the New England Journal Medicine (April 17, 1997) was designed to test the effects of dietary patterns on blood pressure. Rather than use supplements to study single nutrients, the study used whole foods. The diet retained the BP benefits of a vegetarian diet but included enough meat and dairy products to make it palatable and acceptable to the general population. The key findings of this study: that a diet rich in fruits, vegetables and lowfat dairy foods, with reduced saturated and total fat can substantially lower blood pressure. This offers an additional nutritional approach and possible alternative to medication in the treatment of mild hypertension, and possibly prevents or delays medication of borderline HTN. The researchers estimated that if all in the U.S.A. followed the DASH diet and experienced similar results, that coronary artery disease and stroke would be reduced by 15% and 27% respectively, nationwide. This would mean 225,000 fewer heart attacks and 100,000 fewer strokes every year.

The study design included 459 subjects, ages 22 or older, with an average age of 44. About equally divided between men and women, about 2/3 were of racial or ethnic minorities, with 59% being African Americans. All had initial BP less than 160/95 and average baseline BP was 132/85. About 1/3rd had mild HTN (BP 140-159/90-99). The study ran 11 weeks. After an initial 3 week control diet patterned after a typical American diet, subjects were randomized to one of three diets:

1) **Control diet**—typical American diet with 37% calories from fat and low in fruits, vegetables and dairy foods.

2) **Fruit & vegetable diet**—high in fruits and vegetables, similar to control diet, with fewer snacks and sweets.

3) **Combination diet**— high in fruits and vegetables and in lowfat dairy products, with total fat reduced to 27% and saturated fat to 7% of total calories.

All three diets were similar in salt and alcohol content. Calorie intake was also controlled so that subjects maintained their usual body weight. No specialty foods with fat substitutes were used. Fresh, canned and frozen foods were all used.

Compared to the control diet, **the combination diet was most effective, significantly lowering both systolic and diastolic pressure, (mean reduction of 5.5 mm Hg over 3.0 mm Hg).** Reductions in blood pressure were greatest in hypertensive subjects, with a mean reduction of 11.4 mm Hg systolic and 5.5 mm Hg diastolic. The fruit & vegetable diet resulted in about half the magnitude of reduction of the combination diet, speaking well of low fat dairy products, (or of calcium intake). Reductions in BP happened in all ethnic groups, including Caucasians, and among both sexes. Results were noted within 2 weeks and were sustained throughout the study.

OPTIMUM HEALTH DIET PLAN:

Written by one of our editors, Mary Farkas, RD, MS, MA, this diet is a useful place to start for patients with common health problems such as:

1) Irritable Bowel Syndrome (IBS)

2) Gastro-esophageal Reflux Disease (GERD)
3) Diabetes
4) Hyperlipidemia
5) Coronary Artery Disease (CAD)
6) Hypertension (HTN)
7) Obesity
8) Chronic constipation.

This diet plan may be photocopied for use in counseling patients in a medical or allied health setting, but does not substitute for the individual counseling your patient requires. The amounts of food and calorie levels can be adjusted to meet your patient's needs.

There is a paucity of specific nutrition information as regards gastro-intestinal disorders. Gastro-enterologists generally recommend eating a high fiber and/or low fat diet for most of the common, functional GI disorders such as IBS, GERD and constipation. Unless the patient is referred to a Registered Dietitian, specifics of how to change the patient's present offending diet are not communicated by the medical team. Typically the physician will provide lists and meal plans provided by the pharmaceutical companies. Most patients given such lists and meal plans will not optimally change their diet and the GI symptoms persist, necessitating treatment with fiber tablets or phylum, medication, and/or surgery. The dietitian is usually able to ferret out what combination of fibers and foods will resolve the chronic GI problem. For example, if raw vegetables are offending, it may be that cooking them will resolve the problem.

The recent Diabetes Control and complications Trial proved that good glycemic control can and will result from consistency of carbohydrate intake. Typically the physician provides the patient with another pharmaceutical generated "exchange list" and is left on their own for devising (or not) an eating plan which can positively effect their glucose levels. Additionally, the same paucity of information prevails when it comes to cholesterol, triglyceride, and hypertension control. Typically medication is the first line of treatment, when actually medical nutrition therapy is more cost effective for the patient and for society.

Dietitians are trained to view the whole patient, thus recognizing that the patient with IBS may be at risk of, or actually have accompanying diseases such as diabetes, hypertension, hyperlipidemia, CAD, depression or anxiety. The optimum diet for GI disorders will also benefit these other conditions, and vice versa. The foundation the diet is a well-balanced, consistent carbohydrate intake. It has adequate protein, is high in calcium, low in saturated fat, low in refined sugar and overall is moderate in fat. It is plant based, high in phytochemicals, including isoflavones from soy products. This combination of nutritional factors has been shown to treat or help prevent lipid, glucose, and gastro-intestinal disorders, as well as hypertension and obesity. It is also extremely useful for use with patients who are in recovery from alcohol and/or drugs due to the beneficial effects that soluble fibers and consistent carbohydrate intake have on glucose regulation.

DAILY FOOD GUIDE:

1 c. high fiber cereal (130 calories, 1 gram fat, 8 grams fiber, 2-4 grams protein)

3 whole pieces or 3 c. fresh fruit (225 cal, 1 g fat, 9 g fiber, 1 g protein)

1 to 2 cups cooked vegetables (60-120 cal, 1-2 g fat, 4-8 g fiber, 2 g protein)

1 cup raw vegetables (25 cal, 1 g fat, 1 g fiber, 1 g prot)

½ to 1 cup cooked legumes (beans, lentils) or tofu, firm. (100-225 cal, 1-3 g fat, 0*-14 g fiber, 7-14 g protein)

6 to 10 starches (1 st= 1/2 c. potatoes, brown rice, pasta, 1 sl. w/w bread, 1 small corn or w/w flour tortilla) (480-800 cal, 6-8 g fat, 6-15 g fiber, 12-20 g protein)

2 c. non-fat or 1% milk or low sugar yogurt (200-250 cal, 0-5 g fat, 0 g fiber, 20 g prot)

2 to 6 oz. Low fat animal protein (fish, poultry, low fat cheese, seafoood, very lean beef or pork; vegetarians may use dairy, tofu, or legumes) (100-300 cal, 2-18 g fat, 0 g fiber unless vegetarian sources used, 14-42 g protein)

2 tsp. Olive, canola, safflower or sesame oil (89 cal, 9 g fat, 0 g fiber, 0 g protein)

2 Tbsp. Sesame tahini, almond butter, sunflower seed butter or peanut butter (200 cal, 16-18 g fat, 2 g fiber, 8 g protein)

TOTALS: 1600-2355 calories, 38-66 g fat, 30-57 g fiber, 67-112 g protein.

*tofu lacks fiber.

SUGGESTED MEAL PLAN:

Breakfast:
1 cup high fiber cereal
1 sl. whole grain bread with 1 Tbsp. Nut or seed butter
1 cup or 1 piece fresh fruit (fresh preferred over canned)
1 cup non-fat or 1% milk or non-sugar yogurt
Hot beverage of choice (non-sugar)

Lunch: 1 cup or 1 piece fresh fruit
½ to 1 cup brown rice OR pasta OR 1 to 2 sl. whole grain bread OR 1 to 2 small flour or corn tortillas.
½ to 1 cup cooked beans or tofu (OK to use canned beans or bean soups if sodium is not an issue—check with your dietitian or physician).
1 cup raw or cooked vegetables (all dark green leafy vegetables are best)
1 tsp. Oil (see variety recommended above)—use oil to cook, or add to vegetables
Hot or cold beverage of choice (non-sugar)

Snack: (could be added to a meal)
1 piece or 1 cup fresh fruit
1 or 2 sl. whole grain bread with 1 Tbsp. Nut or seed butter

Supper: 2 to 6 oz. Animal (or vegetarian) protein. (recommend: fish, no-skin
Poultry, seafood or game meat; advise beef or lamb < 8 oz. Per week)
1 cup cooked vegetables (emphasize good variety)
1 to 1 ½ cups cooked brown rice OR pasta OR potato
1 tsp. Oil (see variety recommended above)—use oil to cook, or add to vegetables. Suggestion: stir-fry the protein and vegetables using a cooking spray and add 1 tsp. Sesame oil. Add fresh ginger and a splash of soy sauce, and stir till vegetables are crispy done. Serve on a bed of brown rice or noodles).

Snack: (could be added to a meal)
1 cup non-fat or 1% milk OR non-fat yogurt (no sugar)
1 to 2 slices whole grain toast OR t to 2 graham crackers (4 to 8 scored sections of cracker) OR 2 to 6 cups no-oil popcorn.

*This page may be photocopied for patient education purposes, compliments of contributing editor, Mary Farkas, MS, RD, MA. See text for full explanation-- Integrative Medicine, 2nd ed

Evaluation of Popular Diets:
    The Mediterranean diet emphasizes the use of olive oil, pasta, and the traditional salad and main dish preparations of that part of the world. Fish and poultry are more often eaten than beef. As a mono-unsaturated fat, olive oil tends to lower LDL without lowering HDL when compared to the same amount of fat taken in a more saturated form as in the typical American or European diet. The diet is lower in sodium, higher in potassium and antioxidants, and may help prevent arteriosclerosis. (H:C+;143). There is also evidence of decreased cancer risk and decreased overall mortality rates when this diet is followed. (H:C+; 572). However, if one needs to lose excess fat, the typical Mediterranean diet may need modification. The use of native foods such as grapes, (incl. moderate wine) and artichokes have specific health benefits (see under "Herbs and Selected Foods," p. 81).
    Dean Ornish's (and other very low fat) diets, when attention is paid to ensuring adequate nutrient intake, including essential fatty acids, make it possible to prevent and, in many cases, even reverse coronary heart disease, (H:B to C;222-224). The diet for reversal of atherosclerosis and coronary heart disease allows only about 10% of calories from fat—therefore consider supplementation with essential fatty acids. One may supplement as 2 tsp. Of safflower oil (taken PO or applied to the skin). (Dr. Ornish's program that yielded reversal of CAD included a whole treatment package, including smoking cessation).
    Vegetarian diets vary from no animal products whatsoever, (including no dairy products)—the "vegan" diet, to lacto-ovo vegetarian which includes milk and eggs, to diets which include occasional fish or meats. There is very good data from a variety of studies indicating the benefits of the latter diet—one which is plant based and low in fat, with occasional fish or meats, (H:B+; 91, 141). The lacto-ovo vegetarian diet includes the benefits of these studies provided it does not become too high in fat, (e.g. with excess full fat cheese). Some small studies, epidemiological associations and theoretical grounds exists for benefits of the vegan diet over the others, except in infants and small children in whom 2 more essential amino acids are needed than adults, and in whom zinc, iron and calcium status are particularly important for growth and development (104, 141). Calcium and vitamin B-12 may need supplementing, (or use of foods fortified with these nutrients should be considered) in vegan diets. Iron and zinc stores may become depleted—consider diet and/or blood analysis occasionally (see diet analysis below). Vegetarian diets tend to be higher in antioxidant vitamins and phytochemicals. They are associated with living longer and with lower rates of both cancer and heart disease (H:B;91, 141)

The Zone Diet was popularized by Barry Sears' 1995 book entitled, Enter the Zone, A Dietary Road Map To: lose weight permanently, reset your genetic code, prevent disease, achieve maximum physical performance, enhance mental productivity. This diet advocates a strict 40% carbohydrate, 30% protein, and 30% fat intake. It's premise is that Americans are getting fatter because they eat too many carbohydrates, and thus not enough protein and fat, and the high carbohydrate load produces an insulin surge and thus body fat storage. The hallmark of fad diets— fantastic claims (e.g.: reset your genetic code, achieve maximum physical performance, enhance mental productivity, lose weight permanently) is prevalent in his book. The author has strict do's and don'ts for eating, such as the directive to eat 30% of your calories from fat in order to get rid of your fat. It is considered OK to eat a high fat food as long as you "offset" this with enough low-fat protein. Brown rice, wheat bread and potatoes are to be avoided because of their propensity to cause increased insulin production. Protein to carbohydrate ratios are kept to a strict 0.75 with each meal and snack, leading one of our editors to muse that any fat lost could be attributed to spending more time calculating ratios than eating. The diet apparently fails to make a distinction between empty calorie nutrient poor carbohydrates and those that are nutrient rich. For example, high fructose corn syrup soft drinks would be considered of equal value as whole wheat bread. In support of the theories used to construct this diet, Dr. Sears seems to put too much credence on a significantly flawed and unreproducible study published in the Lancet in 1956. This diet has insufficient data to counter the reality that an excess of calories, from any source, will produce an excess of body weight. It may help mobilize people's belief that they can eat better, exercise more, etc.—in a "remembered wellness" effect that may lead to weight loss. However, at this time it does not seem to stand up to scientific scrutiny as an actually effective diet of itself.

"EAT RIGHT FOR YOUR BLOOD TYPE" diet: by naturopathic doctor Peter J. D'Adamo is, in the editor's opinion, an example of taking advantage of the public's ignorance of science in order to make the best seller list. D'Adamo argues that blood type A people cannot digest meat and thus should follow a vegetarian diet. They were the original agrarian grain farmers. Blood type O, the oldest blood type, the original "hunters," should eat meat because their stomach contents are more acidic than blood type A's. Also, the book advises, bananas should be avoided by blood type A's because bananas will interfere with their digestion. Blood type B's (the nomads), should consume dairy products, little meat and no chicken. Blood type AB's (the newest blood type originating approximately 900 A.D.), should consume wheat-free grains, soy products, dairy, seafood, and little meat. D'Adamo maintains that lectins (proteins) in our food cause production of antibodies if the wrong blood type eats the wrong food. He goes on to assert that these antibodies so powerfully disrupt our digestive and immune function that diabetes, hypertension, allergies, and a host of other medical problems ensue. With credulity the public has bought into this. There are blood type chat rooms on the internet, and blood type experts will be happy to answer your questions. In this day and age, when all scientific literature has pointed to the measurable increase in risk and development of much chronic disease from a diet high in saturated fats and low in plant foods, this diet book advises huge numbers of people to eat a meat based, low plant food diet! In the editor's opinion this amounts to the literary equivalent of medical malpractice.

SUGAR BUSTERS! ™ : The newest weight loss book to hit the market is Sugar Busters! ™ Cut Sugar to Trim Fat by H. Leighton Steward, Morrison C. Bethea MD, Samuel Andrews MD and Luis Balart MD. Published by Balantine Books, New York, it was copyrighted in 1995 and 1998. The term "Sugar Busters!" is protected by trademark, an indication that the authors are interested in capitalizing on more than just the sale of this book.

Sugar Busters!™ uses the same pseudo-scientific theory that last year's diet craze book, The Zone Diet used: that eating high glycemic-index starches will create an increase in insulin production, which will lead to obesity. While it is true that eating refined, high glycemic index starches leads to an increase in insulin production, the glycemic index itself has been widely criticized for testing foods individually, which is not how food is generally eaten. When we eat potatoes, white bread, white pasta, corn, beets, carrots (just a few of the forbidden foods) we rarely eat these foods alone; they are almost always part of a mixed meal. The other meal components in toto determine the level of glucose production and thus insulin release. Also, an increase in insulin production, in and of itself, does not lead to obesity. The lack of sufficient physical activity and a surfeit of total food consumed (total surplus calories) leads to obesity. The book does not appear to encourage an increase in physical activity to promote not only weight loss but improved mental and physical health. The book's 14 day meal plan does not contain recommended amounts to be eaten, and the recipes use excessive amounts of fat. For example, one recipe calls for ¾ cup of olive oil, 2 slices of bacon and 1 oz. of cheese to cook portabella mushrooms to serve 2 people!

The book shares a common theme with many recent best selling popular diets—that we have been "hoaxed" by the American nutrition industry. Such sensationalism definitely sells, but at what cost? The glycemic index has been criticized as a tool to create dietary change because the individual foods listed were tested alone, not in the form of a mixed, balanced meal.

Research leading to the glycemic index largely comes from the nutrition "establishment" they are lambasting! Yet it is such research that seems to form the foundation of their book, (while academic criticism of the glycemic index seems to be minimized).

Weight loss diets- see under "Obesity" p. 64-66.

TO SUPPLEMENT OR NOT TO SUPPLEMENT? (See also Nutrition table, p. 112). Seventy percent of people use nutritional supplements at least occasionally. (136).

Who benefits from nutritional supplements? (See also table of herbs and selected foods, p. 81). Among the more frequent valid reasons to take supplements (H:B; 136):

1. Those with low calorie intake—esp. the elderly with decreased appetites or anyone on a weight loss diet, theoretically at least would be expected to benefit from a multiple vitamin & mineral supplement.
2. Lactose intolerant individuals, unless they eat a lot of dark green vegetables and perhaps regular use of almonds or calcium-set tofu, would likely benefit from calcium supplements.
3. Pregnant women (or women who may soon become pregnant), should consider daily folic acid supplements 0.4 mg or 400 micrograms per day.
4. Vegans need B-12 fortification or supplementation
5. Those with specific health problems or needs which have been accurately diagnosed and for which reasonable benefit (compared to risk) exists for the given supplement. Many of these are listed under "systems" in this book, such as the ketogenic diet—listed under Nervous system (Vs seizures), p. 71. Many potentially therapeutic applications of nutrition are summarized by Werbach's Nutritional Influences on Illness, second edition (317).

Who is most likely to be harmed by the use of supplements? (136)

1. Children who accidentally take an overdose of supplements, especially iron supplements, (the #1 cause of childhood death due to poisoning in the USA is accidental iron supplement overdose) (see also ref. 230)
2. Those on prescription medications which interact adversely— the most notable of which is vitamin E's effect on increasing activity of coumadin.
3. Supplementing one nutrient may decrease absorption or utilization of another. For example, calcium (or other mineral) supplements decrease iron absorption.
4. Excess zinc decreases copper stores, immune function, and HDL (good cholesterol) levels.

5. Occasional contaminants of supplements occur—rarely with lethal effects, (e.g.. The eosinophilia - myalgia syndrome associated with contaminated tryptophan; heavy metal contamination of calcium supplements arising from oyster shell or "natural" sources - (136, 319)
6. Theoretically, use of large doses of supplements (above RDA levels) could down-regulate metabolic processes that absorb and store them. Such processes ensure proper absorption, transport, re-cycling and elimination of nutrients. If the patient is habitually ingesting large doses of a nutrient, absorption may be relatively decreased and elimination increased. If the supplements are then suddenly withdrawn, clinical deficiency may soon follow.

Prospective studies on use of nutritional supplements have yielded mixed results:

1. Calcium supplementation was shown effective in alleviating the mood, edema and food craving problems of premenstrual syndrome. (H:B; 470). The study group took 1200 mg of elemental calcium, as calcium carbonate, every day.
2. Beta-carotene supplements in smokers was associated with an increased incidence of lung CA (H:B;4); their use in one large study was associated with increased risk of fatal MI (H:B+;244)
3. Beta-carotene supplements had no effect on incidence of colorectal adenomas (H:B;236).
4. Vitamin E supplements have been associated with decreased risk of coronary artery disease but an increased risk of hemorrhagic stroke, and no overall change in overall mortality rates. (H:A;4, 248).
5. Antioxidant supplements given to prevent cancer have failed or given contradictory results in the first three major clinical trials. (H:D;245).
6. Beta-carotene, Vitamin E and selenium supplements given in an area of China with poor nutrient intake and high incidence of esophageal cancer, decreased death rates due to cancer. (H:B;25)
7. Nutritional supplement use among a cohort of 10,758 persons followed over 13 years, showed overall death rates and death rates due to cancer were essentially the same between users and non-users of supplements. (H:B+;148). This gives credence to the ADA's position of promoting a variety of foods in moderation, with supplements being used only for specific reasons and with dietary assessment. (136).
8. Fish oil supplements—see sixth paragraph down.

Recent data on popular nutritional issues:

- **Antioxidants**– those at increased risk for poor antioxidant intake include the poor, tobacco users, and the elderly (especially the elderly who live alone) (H:B;325). (See also review by Tribble- 297)
- **Cancer prevention** —eat at least 5 servings of fruits and vegetables per day. (H:B;122, 178). Cancer prevention by nutritional means is reviewed by Maberly (178). Eating the recommended amount of fruits and vegetables is associated with practicing other healthy behaviors. (207).
- **Cooked vs. raw fruits and vegetables:** There is abundant evidence that many fruits and vegetables help prevent cancer. But what happens when you cook those fruits and vegetables? In a rigorous study, over 50 fruits and vegetables were tested for efficacy against mutagenic compounds in the lab. Some of the heat stable winners were: blueberries, strawberries, spinach, brussels sprouts and pumpkin. (L:B; 547). Some varieties of apples maintained anti-mutagenic effects when cooked, while others did not.
- **Fluoridation of water**—Recent reviews confirm the efficacy and safety of fluoridation of water to appropriate levels, (H:A; 466, 467)
- **Food vs. supplements**– Do you get the same benefit from supplements as you would from eating the foods from which they were derived? It would appear that in general the food sources are preferable but at least under specific conditions supplements are of benefit. (See above). Haskell and others are studying these issues at Stanford University School of Medicine. The ADA points out that, until proven otherwise, the health benefit of a food does not equal the health benefit of the suspected active ingredient extracted into the form of a supplement.

Fish oil supplements have anti-thrombotic and anti-inflammatory effects (H:B+; 417-423). They have been used effectively in rheumatoid arthritis, HTN and Ig-A nephropathy (H:B-; 418). While moderate fish consumption is associated with decreased mortality due to ischemic heart disease, use of fish oil supplementation has failed to produce the same effect (H:B+; 419). High fish consumption is associated with a trend toward preservation of cognitive function into old age (H:C; 422). There is some concern that fish oil supplements promote LDL peroxidation, especially in diabetics (H:B; 420). There is evidence for an inhibitory

- effect on neoplasm growth and metastasis by these oils (421, 469).
- **Trans fatty acids** are associated with atherogenesis (H:B; 323, 423). "Vegetable shortening" and "partially hydrogenated" oils contain trans fatty acids. Olive or canola oils are preferable to these. (H:B;323). Trans fatty acids were associated with increased risk of breast and colon cancer in a large human study (H:B; 565, 566), though some smaller animal studies suggest little if any effect (A:C; 564).
- **Irradiation of food** for sanitation purposes causes subtle changes similar to those that occur with heating foods or even with natural ripening. These changes appear to have no health consequences. Irradiation of food appears to be both safe and effective as a sanitary measure. (H:A;39).
- **Athletic performance** continues to be a popular reason to take supplements or go on a special diet. In most cases the popularity continues to be greater than the data. Greater knowledge regarding supplements is actually associated with less use of them among high school athletes. (H:C; 183).

Androstenedione is a naturally occurring anabolic steroid which is active "as is" as well as when converted by the body to testosterone. Its use gained notoriety when it became public knowledge that the record-setting baseball player, Mark McGwire used this "nutritional supplement." It may soon be promoted as an aphrodisiac for women, in the form of chewing gum, based on the supposed observation of increased libido in female German athletes who allegedly used this substance.1(591) There are valid concerns, though little data, that androstenedione, like testosterone, may cause liver tumors and accelerate atherosclerosis. Its use in children may stunt height. (562, 555). Similar concerns could be raised for the use of 19-Norandrostenediol and 19-Norandrostenedione. Some body builders and athletes take these compounds with chrysin, which, like other flavonoid compounds, may offer some protective effect on the liver. (L:B; 554).

Chromium was recently found ineffective for "burning fat" or gaining lean muscle mass among weight lifters (H:C+; 175).

Creatine supplements may benefit those who engage in sports which require repetitive sprints—particularly when doing so at the end of already exhausting exercise (H:B;185, 553, 562). Anecdotal reports of GI upset, dehydration and muscle cramps have been reported. (562). The FDA is currently investigating whether the use of creatine supplements is associated with brain tumors and seizures. (562). Typical dosing is a 5 day "loading" period wherein 25 grams per day is ingested, followed by "maintenance" of 5 grams per day.

Carnitine, choline and antioxidant supplements have little if any good controlled scientific data to support their use (H:D to F;145). The possible exception to this may be the use of vitamin E supplements to protect the liver from adverse effects of DHEA (A:C; 561).

DHEA, (dehydroepiandrosterone), is a popular supplement among many persons—not just athletes. There is evidence supporting its effect to promote lean body mass preservation and growth. Its use may alleviate a variety of aging effects, such as muscle wasting, osteoporosis, vaginal atrophy, and insulin resistance. In general the research done in these areas includes both human and animal data, though most studies were small. (557- 560), DHEA is a known hepatocarcinogen in rats—an adverse effect that may be preventable by generous doses of vitamin E. (A:B to C; 556, 561).

Endurance athletes do benefit from high carbohydrate diets and glycogen loading techniques before a race, (if done properly)(H:A; 216). Such athletes may also experience a decreased rate of lactic acidosis—and therefore increased time to exhaustion—by taking dihydroxyacetone and pyruvate supplements before their events (H:B; 552). Iron deficiency may be prevalent enough to warrant screening in endurance athletes, (as may zinc deficiency among vegetarian athletes—preliminary study by Wirth).

OSTEOPATHIC MEDICINE: is a branch of medical care which emphasizes wholistic principles and the practice of "osteopathic manipulative treatment" (OMT). Training for osteopathic physicians includes 4 years of medical school, internship and, usually, a residency program—often done in one of the primary care specialties. After graduation, physicians in this discipline receive the D.O. degree—which is recognized in all 50 states of the U.S. Their "wholistic" training includes conventional western medicine and surgery, along with an emphasis on taking into account the patient's circumstances and lifestyle.

OMT involves massage and musculoskeletal manipulation techniques. There is fairly good evidence of OMT's efficacy in treating low back pain (H:B; 521, 522) and carpal tunnel syndrome (H:C+; 524). It appears to be useful in some cases of dysmenorhea in which pain is felt in the low back (H:C; 520). OMT may also be useful adjunctive treatment of asthma (see ref. 523 and compare with data on massage therapy). OMT has been promoted as effective versus sinusitis, migraine, and other ills, but as yet we have not found relevant studies that evaluate these potential uses.

PROLOTHERAPY: through the use of a series of injections of saline or dextrose in water, (with or without local anesthetic), small injuries are induced at tendon-bone junctions. As the tissue heals, it becomes stronger than before the treatment, and, hopefully, it also heals with a decrease in pain. Prolotherapy is used to treat a variety of orthopedic pain syndromes and for chronic headache cases. Animal data exists to support the basic mechanism of how it works and there are at least two published reports of efficacy in human trials. (A:C; H:D; 484). More studies are warranted since the problems treated are common and can be difficult to manage through other means.

SLEEP: (see also insomnia—p. 64) A very large study conducted in the 1960's suggested increased mortality rates among adults who regularly sleep less than 6 or more than 8 hours per night(H:B; 542). In 1992 Enstrom and colleagues published a classic study which correlated several lifestyle habits with longevity (see "Longevity"—p. 70). According to this study (H:B+; 78), sleeping 7 to 8 hours a night is associated with longevity. A more recent review suggests that 8 to 8.5 hours per night is optimal for adults, and that cutting this short by 1.5 hours results in a 32% decline in daytime alertness! (H:B; 541). Sufficient sleep seems to be important for normal immune system function (H:C; 543).

SPIRITUALITY: see under "SYSTEMS," p. 75.

THERAPEUTIC TOUCH:

Defined differently by different authors, it may include massage or it may specifically refer to a therapy wherein the patient is almost but not actually touched. This latter technique implies some energy transfer through air, which is supposedly detectable and transmittable by therapists. This notion was disproved by Emily Rosa, a scientifically minded 9 year old.(H:B+; 548). The data for benefit with actual massage is very good (H:A-B; see under "Massage Therapy"). As noted, attempts to verify a mechanism for benefit for "almost touching" have either failed or been non-reproducible (H:A; 361, 362, 548).

Apparently because of roots in such religious practices as neopaganism and New Age, the federal government's Equal Opportunities Employment Commission (EEOC) considers TT to be among a number of techniques in which employers may not require employees to participate if it is contrary to their beliefs (587, 588). In the USA, therefore, RNs who object to training in Therapeutic Touch being imposed upon them can invoke the EEOC rule.

Yoga: has relaxant and blood pressure lowering effects (H:B; 15, 451). Improves flexibility and promotes repair of injured muscles (H:B, 448, 449); vs. carpal tunnel syndrome (H:C; 465); supportive treatment in CAD, asthma, insomnia, addictions, and back pain and chronic pain management (H:B to D, 448, 449, 450, 451, 452, 573).

A SYSTEMS APPROACH TO THE POTENTIAL USE OF COMPLEMENTARY THERAPIES

GENERAL CONSIDERATIONS: Please read the "Reason and Caution" section on page 19.

AGING: see "Longevity" (p. 70)

CANCER:

GENERAL PREVENTION:
- **Nutrition: Antioxidants**—data for preventing cancer by the use of unprocessed foods (and spices) high in antioxidants is excellent (H:A); data for the same benefit from extracted antioxidants, minerals or vitamins is poor (178, 245, 268, 297)—Bottom line for now is to emphasize fruits and vegetables as one's best sources of antioxidants. (List of medicinal plant antioxidants-in descending order of strength: hypericum, eleutherococcus, rhodiola, leonurus, aralia, valeriana, echinopanax, schisandra, panax ginseng. L:B; 30). Nutritional supplements with antioxidant and probable preventative value: glutathione and lipoic acid (L:B; A:C; 570, 571). **Foods and spices specifically cited as preventive:** relatively low fat, high vegetable diet (to prevent colon and other cancers)(H:A; 424, 425, 426); cruciferous vegetables (H:B, 317); dark green leafy vegetables (H:B, 317); fruits, nuts and legumes (to prevent cancers) (H:B; 192); soy (incl. tofu)(H:B; 317.); garlic (to prevent stomach CA)(H:B; 301); diets rich in omega-3 fatty acids (fish or green vegetables) (A:B+; 469); whole-grain barley (preventing colon CA)((A:C; H:D); yogurt (preventing breast and colon CA)(H:C-;83); cumin (prevention of gastric CA (A:C; 83); rosemary (to prevent breast CA; A:C; 83); turmeric (A:B; H:C; 83); saffron (A:C-; 83). See also under "lifestyle" – next paragraph. Avoidance of **chlorinated water:** chlorination of water in general prevents a lot of infectious disease but has recently been associated with some increased risk for cancer (especially colon cancer). (H:B; 447).
- **General dietary composition:** see optimum health diet (p. 38-41)

Lifestyle: abstaining from tobacco and xs alcohol (H:A; 348, 370, 371); emphasize dark-green and yellow vegetables in the diet while avoiding pickled or smoked foods (H:B; 317); vegetarian (or nearly vegetarian) diet (H:B; 317); moderate exercise (H:C; 348); avoid overcooked beef or pork (applies to grilling or frying) (H:C; 438); resolve or get rid of anger and other negative emotions through non-destructive means (H:C-; 434); see also lifestyle habits listed under "longevity" (p. 70).

- **Herbs:** garlic (prevention of stomach CA)(H:B; 301); glucomannan (preventing lung CA)(A:C-; 83); turmeric (A:B; H:C); saffron (A:C-); clove (post toxin exposure)(A:C-; 83); perilla (preventing colon CA)(A:C; 83); rosemary (preventing breast CA)(A:C; 83); carefully selected mushrooms probably have preventive value—esp. Lentinus (Shiitake), Pleurotus, Auricularia, Flammulina (enokitake), Tremella and Grifola (maitake) (see review by Chang (47); see under table on Herbs and Selected Foods, p. 81. See also list of antioxidants— 2 paragraphs up.

TREATMENT OF CANCERS:

General considerations: Remember that rigorous, well-funded research is leading to significant advances in "orthodox" cancer treatment. Alternative therapies may be in a position to claim effectiveness when patients recover yet, through the usual disclaimers, blame the disease, patient or the medical establishment when patients fail to recover. This "heads I win, tails you lose" stratagem aside, those clinicians and patients facing cancer may wish to compare serious but contrasting sources of information, then work out a "integrative" plan. Cooperation between oncologist, patient and primary care provider is needed. Consider these sources:

1) Social and spiritual support in a way appropriate to the patient, (see ref. 407).
2) Michael Lerner's book, Choices in Healing, (The MIT press, 1996), does an admirable job of presenting conventional and alternative treatment options for patients.
3) For an excellent review of nutrition and cancer, see Werbach's Nutritional Influences on Illness (ref. 317). Most data supports the emphasis of a vegetarian or nearly vegetarian diet to prevent many cancers, but data supporting such a diet to treat cancer once it is diagnosed is grossly lacking. The use of therapeutic diets may delay the use of effective conventional treatment and thus do harm. (596).

4) For excellent reference data on herbs that have anti-neoplastic activity, see Boik's text, Cancer and Natural Medicine (ref. 369). Boik's good judgment is refreshing in that he documents the research on many herbs with potential benefit, while giving credit to the better-studied effects of chemotherapy on the more common cancers.

There seems insufficient data at this time to recommend herbs over orthodox therapy. Even the data to advise integrating the use of herbs with orthodox methods is modest in most cases, at least in English literature. More quality research is needed.

5) Reports from the American Cancer Society and other reliable patient education and data base sources (see "Favorite Web Sites"—p. 56)

6) A consult from "Healing Choices"—a non-physician led research service which, for about $275, will take a detailed history of a given patient, research the relevant "alternative therapy" options, and send a report back in a timely manner. Unfortunately, at the expense of risking their credibility, this service comes with advertisements for literature that appears to portray chemotherapy research as a greed-driven conspiracy. The editors would welcome independent evaluations of this service. To obtain a consult request form from Healing Choices, call (USA); 718-636-4433, e-mail : equinox@walrus.com

7) Reports on cancer treatment quackery from the National Council for Reliable Health Information: web: www.ncahf.org

Treatment of specific cancers arising from specific organs: (plant names refer to their use as herbs or extracts in therapeutic amounts in research designs, that is, not in homeopathic amounts).

- **Bladder:** mistletoe (commercial extract only)(H:C; 316).
- **Breast:** inclusion in support groups improved survival (H:B; 375, 376); moderate exercise improved quality of life & increased natural killer cell activity (H:C;232); yew extracts (paclitaxol)(H:C; 83); Catharanthus roseus (the plant source of vinblastine and vincristine)(A:C, 369); gossypium (A:C; 69, 369); Isatis tinctoria (A:C; 369); juglans regia (A:C; 369); mistletoe extract (H:C; 316); oldenlandia diffusa (H:C; 369); shiitake mushroom (H:C-; 316); vitamin E vs. Estrogen receptor negative breast CA (L:C;149, 299); rheum officinale and rheum tanguticum (A:C; 69, 369)
- **Cervix:** Arisaematis (Arisaema consanguineum) (H:C; 369); Brucea javanica (H:C; 369); Crotalariae sessiliflorae (H:C; 369); oldenlandia diffusa (H:C; 369); ginseng (panax)(H:D; 69, 369).
- **Choriocarcinoma** (and lesser forms of trophoblastic neoplasm): catharanthus roseus (H:B; 69); trichosanthes kirilowii (H:B; 369)

Colon: Shiitake mushroom extract (lentinan IV)(increases T-cell function)(H:C-; 83); Crotalariae sessiliflorae – vs. rectal CA (H:C; 369); echinacea (H:D; 83); oldenlandia diffusa (vs rectal

- CA)(H:C; 369); (green tea appears to have preventive value)(H:C; 83).

- **Gastric:** houttuynia cordata (H:C; 369); polistes mandarinus (H:C?; 369); shiitake mushroom (H:C; 316).

- **Hepatic:** mylabris phalerata (A:C; 369); siberian ginseng (eleutherococcus)(H:D; 69, 381); cascara (L:C; 83); polistes mandarinus (H:C?; 369); sophora subprostrata (A:C; 369)

- **Leukemia:** Isatis tinctoria (H:C; 369); manis pentadactyla (H:C; 369); echinacea (A:C; 83); cascara (extracts)(A:C; 83); cordyceps (mushroom or extract)(L:B; 48); Crotalariae sessiliflorae (A:C; 369); oldenlandia diffusa (A:C; 369); ginseng (panax)(H:C-; 69, 316, 369); tripterygium wilfordii (A:C; 369)

- **Lung:** Cordyceps sinensis (H:C, 369); mistletoe extract (carefully given under expert supervision)(H:C; 83, 316); seaweed extract (H:C; 316).
- **Lymphoma:** mistletoe extract (H:C; 316).

- **Melanoma:** yew extract (paclitaxol)(H:B-; 83); mistletoe extract (H:C; 316); Dichroa febrifuga (A:C; 369); yucca (A:D+; 83); gossypium (A:C; 69, 369); rheum officinale and rheum tanguticum (A:C; 69, 369).

- **Oral:** turmeric (H:C-; 316).

- **Ovary:** yew extract (paclitaxol)(H:B-; 83)

- **Sarcomas:** oldenlandia diffusa (H:C; 369); aloe vera (A:C; 316); shiitake mushroom (A:C; 316).

- **Skin:** Crotalariae sessiliflorae (H:C; 369)

- **Uterine:** oldenlandia diffusa (A:C; 369)

SUPPORTIVE CARE OF CANCER PATIENTS:
- **vs nausea and vomiting:** if orthodox measures fail, consider marijuana (PO-Marinol; smoked where legal)(H:B; 83) or acupuncture (H:B-; 234, 309).
- **vs anxiety** (and may help immune system?): music (H:B;251, 281); art (H:D;164); support groups (H:B; 375, 376)
- **to alleviate decreasing wbc** during chemotherapy or radiotherapy: echinacea (H:C+;50, 235); music (H:D; 281)
- **to protect GI tract vs radiotherapy** damage: glutamine-supplemented polymeric or elemental diet (ref. 41); eleutherococcus (H:C; 69).
- **to protect vs. Renal toxicity in cisplatin-treated** patients: silibinin (A:B; 29)
- **to increase survival:** support groups (H:B; 375, 376)
- **to improve quality of life:** moderate exercise (H:C; ref.)(caution- xs exercise suppresses immunity- H:A; 214)

HERBS AND NUTRITIONAL SUPPLEMENTS WITH AT LEAST SOME POSITIVE EVIDENCE FOR BENEFICIAL EFFECTS IN TREATING CA:
(see also above under specific organ sites) bioflavonoids (specifically quercetin, myricetin & silymarin; L:B;70); eleutherococcus (A:C; H:D; 83); taheebo (Pau D'Arco)(H:C; 301)(side effects limit dose to sub-therapeutic levels); alpinia (A:C-; 83); burdock (A:C-; 83); celery extracts (A:C; 83); cordyceps sinensis (L:B; 161-2); garlic (A:C; 83, 316); gotu kola (L:D; 83); mace (A:C; 83); honey (A:D-; 83); maitake mushroom extract (204); melatonin (H:C; 83); noni (morinda citrifolia)(A:C-; 128-9); primrose oil (A:C; 83); propolis (A:C; 83); royal jelly (A:D; 83); fenugreek (A:C-; 301); asparagus (L:C-; 83); cat's claw (H:D; 83); chaparral (H:D; 301—caution re: one case of severe liver toxicity noted); yarrow (A:C-; 83); turmeric (H:D-; 83); saffron (A:C-; 83). The CRC Handbook of Medicinal Herbs mentions over 200 herbs with at least traditional records supporting their use against cancer (69).

CARDIOVASCULAR SYSTEM:
anemia: ginseng (H:D?; 301)
angina: see also coronary artery disease; ammi (requires careful monitoring for eye & liver toxicity)(H:B; 83); hawthorn (H:C; 301, 406); musk (H:C; 83)
coronary artery disease: very low fat diet(10% of calories—possibly with supplemented essential fatty acids) + lifestyle modification (achieves reversal of CAD in significant number of patients under supervision)(H:B; 222-225); hawthorn (H:B; 83, 406); eleutherococcus (A:C; 83); ginseng (H:C?; 301); beta-carotene supplements (and perhaps vitamin E supplements) gave no benefit and actually were associated with increased risk of fatal MI (H:B+; 244).
Vs. connective tissue breakdown (aneurysms, etc.): pycnogenol (A:C; 83).

CHOLESTEROL PROBLEMS:

THERAPY	TOT. CHOL	LDL (BAD)	HDL (GOOD)	TRIGL	SAFETY	REF.
ammi			↑		limited	316 (H:C)
avocado		↓			good	83 (H:B)
barley	↓	↓	may ↓		good	83 (H:C)
brewer's yeast	↓	↓	↑	no Δ	good	317 (H:C-)
carrot	↓				good	317
cascara	↓					83 (A:C)
evening primrose oil	↓				good	316(H:B)
exercise	↓	sl. ↓	↑	↓	good	216 (H:A)
fenugreek	↓					316(H:C)
flax seeds		↓	no Δ			83 (H:C?)
garlic	↓	↓	sl. ↑		good	316(H:A-)
ginseng	↓	↓	↑?		good	316 (H:D+)
glucomann.	↓		no Δ			83 (H:B)
guggal	↓	↓	sl. ↑			316 (H:B)
maitake	↓		no Δ	↓	good	158 (A:C)
monascus	↓	↓			good	83 (H:A)
oats	↓				good	317 (H:C)
pectin		↓	no Δ	↓	good	316 (H:B+)
perilla	↓					83 (A:C)
plantain	↓				good	83 (H:B-)
safflower oil	↓	↓	no Δ	no Δ	good	83 (H:C)
saffron (spice)	↓			↓	OK in mod.	83 (A:C)
shiitake mushroom	↓				good	83(H:C?)
wine (red)			↑		OK in mod.	83 (H:B)
yogurt	↓				good	83 (H:C)

congestive heart failure: hawthorn (H:B; 38, 406); cinnamon (increases atrial natriuretic factor which leads to diuresis)(A:D; 83); digitalis (narrow therapeutic window)(H:A-; 83)
dysrhythmias: chicory (extracts)(A:C-; 83, 301); devil's claw (A:C-; 83); digitalis (narrow therapeutic window)(H:A; 83); horehound (H:D; 301); quinine (H:A; 83)
edema: bilberry (A:B-; 83)
hypertension: hawthorn (H:B+; 83, 301); regular exercise (H:B+; 216); garlic (H:B; 301); DASH diet (H:B+; 540, see p. 37); yoga (H:B?; 15); look for and correct obstructive sleep apnea when present (H:B+; 544-546); alpinia (A:C; 83): barberry (H:D; 301); carrot oil (A:C; 83); cat's claw (A:B; 83); celery (extracts)(A:C; 83); devil's claw (A:B; 83); ginseng (H:C-?; 301); guar gum (H:C; 83); yellow root (H:C-; 83); yucca (H:D; 83).
hypotension: herbs, etc. that tend to raise BP: ephedra (may cause dysrhythmias)(H:A; 301); ginseng (H:D; 69).
ischemic heart dz: garlic (H:B+; 300, 406); coenzyme Q (A:C; 83); acupuncture A:B+; 533); fumitory (A:C-; 83)
myocardial infarction: to prevent MI and to improve post MI prognosis: screen for and treat depression (H:A; 14, 93, 238); garlic (H:B; 301).
oxygen diffusion: to increase oxygen diffusion in plasma: saffron (as a spice; avoid large doses)(L:B; H:D+; 83)
peripheral vascular disease: (incl. Raynaud's dz, vaso-occlusive dz, etc.): ginkgo (H:B; 83, 301); pycnogenol (H:C; 83); squill (narrow therapeutic window)(A:B; H:C; 83)
platelet aggregation inhibitors ("blood thinners"): garlic (H:A-; 83); ginkgo (H:D; 249); guarana (H:C-; 83); primrose oil (H:C; 83); wine (H:C+; 83)
prevention of CV dz: do not smoke (H:A; 90, 91, 378, et al.); exercise (decreases risk of primary & secondary cardiac events)(H:A; 169); dietary antioxidants (associated with foods: H:B; with supplements: H:D; 297); increase dietary folate (or folic acid supplements?) to help decrease homocysteine levels (see nutrient table, p. 116); hopes/desires being fulfilled (H:B; 407; see also Proverb 13:12 in the Bible); garlic (H:B; 301); vegetarian diet (H:B; 378, 379, 380); prevent anger and/or handle it well (H:C; 315, 407); specifically for women: optimize social support and prevent or treat chronically negative emotions (H:B; 37, 407); folate (H:C; 303); guggal (to decrease cholesterol)(H:C-; 83); frequent consumption of nuts (H:C+; 92).
post phlebitis syndrome: ginkgo (H:C; 83)
causes increased heart rate: ephedra (also may cause dysrhythmias)(H:A; 301)
causes vasoconstriction: butcher's broom (H:C; 301 p. 65)
vasoprotective (vs HTN induced xs permeability): bilberry (H:C; A:B; 83)

varicose veins: horse chestnut (careful use of standard extracts)(H:C+; 300, 316); butcher's broom (PO)(H:C-; 83); gotu kola (H:C+; 83); witch hazel (PO)(A:D; 301)

DENTAL:

ANESTHETIC (VS PAIN): TENS (transcutaneous electrical nerve stimulation) (H:B+; 549-551); cloves (esp. topical use of oil)(H:A; 83); kava kava (H:C; 83)

vs. Dental anxiety: biofeedback (and other relaxation techniques)(H:B; 77, 407)

CARIES PREVENTION: vanilla (H:D; 83); grape seed & its extracts (L:C; 83)

"DRY SOCKET": clove (esp. oil)(H:A; 83); propolis (H:C; 83); peru balsam (H:C-; 83)

GINGIVITIS: neem oil (H:C-; CI-infants; 83)

PERIODONTAL DZ: folic acid (H:A; 317); other vitamins & minerals to replace deficiencies when present (H:A; 317); licorice root (H:C-; 316); gotu cola (H:C-; 316); calendula (H:D?; 83)

PLAQUE: bloodroot (H:A; 83); acacia (esp. preventative)(H:C; 83)

TMJ & MASTICATORY MYOFASCIAL PAIN: alternative treatments reviewed by Wright and dos Santos (ref.)

DERMATOLOGY:
acne: high fiber, low fat, low simple sugar diet (H:B+; 317); brewer's yeast (H:D; 317); tea tree (H:D; 301)
antiseptic: tea tree (H:C; 301)
baldness: correction of nutritional deficiencies when present (H:B; 317); fenugreek (A:C; 301); remember to check thyroid status (orthodoxy).
bedsores: myrrh (topical)(H:C; 301)
burns: aloe (H:C-; 83)
cancer of the skin: bloodroot (H:C-; A:B; 83); see also "melanoma" and "skin" under "Cancer."
chapped lips: calendura (H:C; 301)
connective tissue protectant: pycnogenol (A:C; 83; theorized to protect vs. aging of skin)

vs dandruff: burdock (topical; H:C-; 83); quillaia (topical only)(H:D; 83); red squill (topical)(H:D; 83)
DIETARY EFFECTS ON SKIN DISEASES: see ref. 363.
dry skin: avocado (oil)(L:B; H:C; 83)
eczema: primrose oil (H:D; 83 & 301); stress management and treatment of other psychological aspects (see review by Cotterill- ref. 58)
vs fleas: tea tree (H:C-?)
vs frostbite: aloe (H:C-; 83)
vs fungal skin or nail infections: clove (esp. topical use of the oil)(H:C; 83); tea tree (H:D—by inference; see table of herbs and selected foods).
hand cleaner: grape seed oil (H:C-; 83)
insect bites (to relief discomfort from): topical witch hazel (H:D; 65)
insect repellent: rosemary (L:C; 83)
poison oak/ ivy (topical treatment): aloe (H:D; 83); plantain leaves (crushed)(H:D; 83)
psoriasis: may clear with elimination diet (e.g.: no red meat, no dairy, some or even all grains may be excluded)(H:C-; 220); ammi (H:C-; 83; caution re: eye & liver side effects esp. with oral use); capsaicin (topical)(H:C; 316); milk thistle extract (silymarin)(H:C; 316); feverfew (H:D; 83); gotu kola (H:C-; 83); juniper (H:C-; 83)
sunscreen: cascara (H:C; 83)
vitiligo: ammi (H:C; 83; caution esp. with oral use); St. John's wort (topical & oral use of extracts)(H:C; 83)
wound healing (topical treatments): angelica (L:B; A:B; 83); calendula (A:C; 83); echinacea (H:C; 301); peru balsam (H:C-; 83); propolis (H:C-; 83)

DIGESTIVE SYSTEM:

alcoholic liver dz: (see also cirrhosis & hepatitis): primrose oil (H:C-; 83)

anxiety (over having endoscopy procedures): self-selected music tapes (H:C+; 360)

antispasmodic: chamomile (H:B; 301); calamus (esp. American strain)(H:C; 301); savory (L:B; H:C-; 83); sage (A:C; 83); raspberry (tea)(H:D; 301); garlic (high dose)(H:C; 301); fennel (avoid oil extracts)(A:B; 301)

bile excretion stimulators: artichoke (H:B; 83); boldo (H:B-; 83)

cholera: barberry (H:C; 83)

cirrhosis: milk thistle (H:B-; 83 & 301)

constipation: apples (H:C; 83); cascara (H:A; 83); glucomannan (konjac)(H:B; 83); senna (H:A; 301); wheat bran; cooked dark green leafy vegetables.

digestive aid: devil's claw (stimulates appetite)(H:D; 301); gentian (H:B; 301); ginger (H:C; 301); horehound (H:D; 301); parsley (H:C; 301); peppermint (may worsen GERD or cholecystitis)(H:B; 301)

diarrhea: oral rehydration salt solution (conventional care but often forgotten—1/2 tsp. Salt plus 2 Tbsp. Sugar per 8 to 12 ounces clean water; sip almost continuously.) (usual care); agrimony (H:B; 83, 406); goldenseal (bourberine is active ingredient & is sold separately)(H:B; 316); Oregon grape root (also contains bourberine)(H:B; 316); raspberry (tea)(H:C; 301); acidophilus (H:D; 83); apples (H:C; 83); betony (H:C-; 83); bilberry (H:C; 83): cinnamon (A:C-; 83): savory (L:B; H:C-; 83); yogurt (vs antibiotic-induce diarrhea)(H:D-; 83)

vs xs gas: charcoal (H:C; 83); fennel (avoid oil extract)(H:B; 301); lovage (H:D?; 301); consider lactose intolerance (usual care).

gastric emptying: white wine (increases rate of gastric emptying but may also worsen GERD)(H:C; 83)

GERD: remember to avoid high fat foods, etoh, nicotine, coffee and peppermint (usual care); licorice root (use of deglycerinized licorice is probably safer)(H:D; 316); barberry (H:D; 301); see also optimum health diet—p.38. Consider checking for B12, iron and calcium deficiency in patients on chronic H-2 blockade.

hemorrhoids: butcher's broom (H:D?; 301); myrrh (H:C; 301); St John's wort (H:D?; 301); peru balsam (H:C-; 83)

hepatitis: milk thistle (H:B-; 83 & 301); ganoderma (mushroom)(vs Hepatitis B:171)aloe (PO or IV)(A:C; 83); high-protein, low-fat diet (usual care).

hunger: peppermint (delays hunger for a brief time)(H:B; 301)

vs inflammatory bowel disease: quercetrin (A:C-; 96).

irritable bowel syndrome: decrease fat and simple sugars in diet (H:B; 317); Chinese herbal medicine (standard preparation of several herbs and individualized selection of herbs by experienced practitioner are both effective) (H:B; 463); increase fiber in diet (H:C; 317); chamomile (H:B; 406); peppermint (H:C; 83); plantain (psyllium fiber)(H:C+; 83); dandelion (H:D; 83).

laxatives: senna (H:A; 83); aloe (PO—very strong)(H:A; 83); fo-ti (H:B; 83 & 301); hibiscus (mild effect)(H:C; 301); yellow dock (H:C?; 301)

liver protectives: (hepatoprotective): artichoke (H:D; 83); carrot oil (A:C; 83); mace (A:C; 83); milk thistle (H:A; 83); turmeric (A:A; H:C; 83)

nausea & vomiting: acupuncture (H:B; 309); acupressure (volar aspect of wrist—"P6" site; H:B; 85); (see 318); marijuana (H:B; 83)

peristalsis (ways to increase peristalsis): (see also constipation & laxatives): garlic (low dose)(H:C; 301)

poisoning: charcoal (H:A; 83)

peptic ulcer dz: licorice root (preferably as deglycerinized)(H:A; 316); high fiber diet (H:C; 317); cabbage (H:C-; 317); alpinia (seeds)(A:C; 83); calendula (A:D?; 83); chamomile (A:C; 83); clove

(A:C-; 83); fenugreek (A:C-; 301); ginseng (esp. preventive)(A:B; 83); honey (vs H. pylori)(H:C; 83); myrrh (H:C; 301); St. John's wort (vs gastritis)(H:D?; 301). Consider checking for vitamin B-12, iron and calcium deficiency in patients who chronically use H-2 blockers.

worms: cucurbita (pumpkin) seeds (H:C; 83)

EAR, NOSE AND THROAT: (See also INFECTIOUS DISEASE and RESPIRATORY headings)

- **versus the common cold:** see under pharyngitis below. Also, consider trying chicken noodle soup (H:D; 83).
- **soothing mucous membranes** (demulcent): tragacanth (H:C-; 83)
- **hearing problems:** ginkgo (may be useful when problem is due to vascular dz involving the ear)(H:C; 83)
- **oral mucosal sores:** goldenseal (H:C; 301)
- **recurrent otitis media:** xylitol-containing chewing gum (inhibits strep pneumonia—moderately effective)(H:B; 304)
- **pharyngitis:** echinacea and zinc lozenges may have both symptomatic and anti-infective benefit (H:B; 301)(zinc mainly vs common viral pharyngitis); the following have data supporting symptomatic relief: acacia gum (H:C; 83); agrimony (H:C-; 83); betony (H:D; 301); bilberry (H:C; 83); coltsfoot (H:B; 83); hyssop (H:D; 83); karaya gum (H:C-; 83); marsh mallow root (H:C-; 301); mullein (H:C; 301 & 83); myrrh (H:C; 301); savory (H:C; 301); slippery elm (extract in lozenges)(H:C-; 83); storax (H:D; 83)
- **sinusitis:** pineapple stem extract (bromelain)(caution re: GI adverse effects)(H:C-; 69, 316).
- **tinnitus:** ginkgo (H:C; 301); acupuncture (H:C; 531).
- **vertigo:** ginkgo (H:C; 83); homeopathic preparation—"Vertigoheel" (H:C; 464).

ENDOCRINE SYSTEM:

DIABETES MELLITUS:
- **Lifestyle:** regular exercise (H:B; 310);
- **Nutrition:** high fiber diet low in simple sugars, (unrefined diet) (usual care); consistent carbohydrate diet (see optimum health diet—p. 38); chromium supplementation may help some (H:C+; 186, 468).

Herbs/Specific foods: glucomannan (H:C+; 83); fenugreek (A:B; H:C; 83); ginseng (H:C; 83; 301); guar gum (esp. AODM)(H:C; 83); gymnema (A:A; H:C-; 83); primrose oil (vs

Systems Approach

diabetic neuropathy)(H:C; 83); artichoke (H:D; 83); eleutherococcus (A:C+; H:D; 83); lavender (vs AODM; A:C+; H:D; 83); neem (A:C; H:D; 83); tragacanth (H:D; 83); dandelion leaves (A:C; 83); horehound (A:C-; 83); Juniper (A:C; 83); myrrh (A:D+; 83); silymarin (from milk thistle)(used in cirrhotic diabetics—cautiously and in experimental protocols)(H:C+; 308)

- **acupuncture** (vs. diabetic neuropathy): 532).

ENDOCRINE CAPACITY ENHANCEMENT: exercise (H:B; 310)

ENDOCRINE WITHDRAWL: black cohosh (H:D+; 83)

MINERALOCORTICOID EFFECT: bayberry (H:C?; 301)

PROLACTIN: vs. Hyperprolactinemia: chaste tree (H:C-; 83)

GASTROINTESTINAL (SEE DIGESTIVE SYSTEM)
GENERAL & MISCELLANEOUS:

- **anemia:** alpinia (A:D; 83)
- **alcohol related illnesses:** vs alcoholism: art tx (H:C-; 111; 98); acupuncture— apparently no difference from placebo (H:C+; 36); vs alcoholic liver dz: primrose oil (H:C-; 83)
- **vs allergies** (see also immune system): saw palmetto (A:C-; 83)
- **anti-inflammatory:** butcher's broom (A:C; 83); calendula (A:C-; 83); chamomile (A:B; 83); chicory (A:C-; 83); fenugreek (A:C-; 83); gentian (H:C?; 301); gotu kola (H:C?; 301); myrrh (A:C; 83); saw palmetto (A:C-; 83); woodruff (A:C-; 83)
- **anti-oxidants** (free radical scavengers): garlic (H:A-; 83); ginkgo (H:A-; 83); milk thistle (H:A-; 83); pycnogenol (H:B; 83); turmeric (A:A; H:B; 83); red wine (& grape juice)(H:B-; 83); alchemilla (H:C; 83); allspice (L:C; 83); cumin (A:C-; 83); grape seed (L:C; 83); melatonin (L:B-; 83); propolis (A:B; 83); rosemary (L:C; 83); sage (L:B-; 83).
- **aphrodisiacs:** summer savory (H:D-; 83); yohimbe (H:D; 83); testosterone (orthodoxy)(PO, IM or dermal)
- **athletic performance** enhancers (ergogenic aids): creatine (for repetitive sprints)(H:C; 185); octacosanol (wheat germ extract)(H:D; 83); see also p. 48-49.
- **chronic fatigue syndrome:** dietary analysis & manipulation (H:C; 110)
- **death/dying:** (see also related problems—nausea & vomiting under Digestive System; Pain; Spirituality, etc.): music therapy (H:C; 259)

-edema: (see also diuretics under Urinary system); ginseng (H:D; 301)
fever: burdock (H:C-; 83)
general well-being: biorhythms managed well (lifestyle)(H:A; 154); exercise (in moderation)(H:A; 310); love (H:B;112); remembered wellness effect, (or placebo effect)—relevant up to about 80% of the time (H:B+; 407); see also spirituality (p. 75) and optimum health diet (p.38).
insomnia: relaxation techniques (progressive muscle relaxation, biofeedback, meditation, or autogenic training)(H:A; 409); valerian (H:B; 83 & 301); acupuncture (H:B-; 172); lavender (aroma tx)(H:C-; 83); light tx (also effective vs jet lag)(H:A; 32, 72); melatonin (H:B-; 83); music tx (H:C-; 199); St. John's wort (H:C?; 301); exercise early in the day & avoid vigorous exercise in the evening or night (usual care)
insect repellent: garlic (H:C?; 372); neem oil (CI in small children)(H:C; 83); lavender (topical)(H:C-; 83)
jet lag: light tx (H:B; 32); melatonin (H:B; 83)
leg cramps: vitamin E (400 IU per day)(H:B; 317); quinine (caution re: thrombocytopenia)(H:B; 83).
libido decreasing (to decrease libido—opposite of aphrodisiacs): winter savory (H:D-; 83)
muscle relaxants (smooth muscle): lavender (A:C; 83); peppermint (H:C; 83)
OBESITY:

- **general information:** obesity is the # 2 cause of death in the USA (smoking is # 1)(187). A popular delusion that leads to failed attempts to lose weight is the notion that: "If giving a nutrient supplement to people who are deficient in it helps them lose weight, then giving that same supplement to most overweight people will also help them lose weight." For weight loss of about 100 or more pounds, surgical approaches have the best documented success (H:A; 217)
- **best diets:**
  1. individualized diet designed for (& with) you by a RD nutritionist
  2. Optimum Health Diet (described by Mary Farkas, RD, MA, MS) (see p.38-41).
  3. high fiber, low fat vegetarian (or nearly vegetarian) diet (avoiding full fat cheese)
  4. Pritikin diet (requires attention to essential fatty acid intake).
  5. Dean Ornish's general diet (the heart disease reversal diet by Dr. Ornish requires attention to essential fatty acid intake)
  6. Weight Watchers

- **herbs or food products that may assist in fat loss:** high fiber diet or fiber supplements; guar gum (H:D; 83); primrose oil (H:D; 83); vanilla (improves satiety)(H:C-; 83); protein foods (improves satiety).
- **review of over the counter (without prescription) weight loss products:**
    1. Acutrim ®, Dextrim®, and others—incl. Oral sprays containing phenylpropanolamine: (H:B- short term efficacy): These medications have shown modest short term effect, with recommended use limited to 1 week to at the most 3 months. They may be hazardous to those with heart, BP or vascular disease.
    2. Ephedra (Ma huang): (H:C); similar precautions as with phenylpropanolamine. (Banned in some states because of medical and possibly addictive risks—related to amphetamines)
    3. Aspartame (Equal®): (H:B) occasional reports of headache.
    4. Aroma therapy: (H:D-) (Little scientific data found—we welcome any for review in this new area)
    5. Cybergenics Quick Trim®: (H:C): for a few of the ingredients we found quality supportive evidence for at least a modest effect. This and many products contain chromium for which the best study we found suggested no efficacy. Many other ingredients included for which we found no scientific data.
    6. Diet Fat Burner®: (H:D)
    7. Chinese Herbs: (H:C-) some published studies, generally small and sub-optimal in design, support use. Reports of serious CV and renal side effects have been made. Caution or waiting for more data advised.
    8. Olestra®(H:C-); may cause xs gas.
    9. Se Quester ®(3 products): The first: fiber (H:B), theoretically some may experience xs gas; the second: phenylpropanolamine (H:B)—see precautions as for Acutrim®; the third: (chromium + carnitine): (H:D-) – little good data & includes negative data.
    10. Ultralean Herbal Weight Loss Plan®: (by use of product itself: H:D; when included with advised calorie restriction + exercise: H:B) Some diuretic herbs included. Little scientific data on several ingredients found.

review of best prescription weight loss meds: (H:A-; 101, 114, 313, 314) With the conservative but reasonable withdrawl of Redux® (d-fenfluramine) and the associated disinterest in "Fen-Phen" (d,l - fenfluramine + phentermine), we are awaiting more research. Some clinicians are using fluoxetine plus or minus phentermine on inference from fair data (H:C), though safety is again questionable. Sibutramine (Meridia) appears to have moderate benefit without the risks associated with Redux.

Weight table for those who may be candidates for prescription medical approach: (noted as follows: height in feet & inches : minimum weight (lbs) to qualify with other risk factors—minimum weight to qualify without other risk factors) (BMI of 27 and 31 kg/m^2, respectively, with risk factors such as DM, HTN or hyperlipidemia):

Height	Weight	Height	Weight
4 ft, 10 in	129-143 lbs	5'9"	183-203
4'11"	134-148	5'10"	188-209
5'0"	138-153	5'11"	193-215
5'1"	143-158	6'0"	199-221
5'2"	147-164	6'1"	204-227
5'3"	152-169	6'2"	210-233
5'4"	157-175	6'3"	216-240
5'5"	162-180	6'4"	222-246
5'6"	167-186	6'5"	227-253
5'7"	172-191	6'6"	233-259
5'8"	177-197	6'7"	239-266

occupational medicine:
- general **work site health appraisal:** AT&T Health Audit is a standard appraisal mentioned by Scofield (262); should include social ecological analysis with consideration of work place environment
- cost-effective **health promotion:** those built in to normal routine are most cost effective (e.g.: walking or cycling to & from work)(H:C; 269)
- **shift work:** light tx (H:C; 72)

pain: relaxation training (H:A; 218, 407); biofeedback (H:B-; 218); hypnotherapy (H:B; 218 & 137); music tx (H:B-; 219); noni (morinda citrifolia)(A:C; 331)

vs radiation: echinacea (A:C; 83); eleutherococcus (L:C; A:C-; 83); pectin (vs GI source of radiation)(H:C; 83)

vs stress: eleutherococcus (A:C; H:C-; 83); ginseng (A:B; H:D; 301); withania (A:C-; 83)

sweating: increases sweating: linden flowers (H:C; 301)

vs toxins: clove (inhibits carcinogenesis)(A:C-; 83); vs amanita mushroom poisoning (and perhaps liver toxins in general?)- milk thistle (esp. IV extracts)(H:A; 83)

vs vertigo: ginkgo (H:C+; 83); ginger (H:C-; 301)

Ach agonist
- methacholine – emergency tx of glaucoma
- carbachol
- bethanechol – GI + GU atony
- pilocarpine – glaucoma

Anticholinesterases
- edrophonium – IV test for MG, supravent tachycardia
- neostigmine – test for MG + anticholinergic OD
- physostigmine – crosses BBB ∴ atropine antidote
- pyridostigmine – Tx for MG

Muscarinic Antagonist
- atropine – eye dilation for examination
- scopolamine – bronchodilator

Ganglionic blockers
- trimethaphan – HTN crisis

Sympathetic agonist
- ephedrine α + β action, like amphetamine but no CNS effect
- phenylephrine – α₁ – nasal decongestion

β2 agonists – bronchodilation resistant to COMT
- metaproterenol
- albuterol
- terbutaline

β2 stimulation = bronchial relaxation

α₁ antagonists
- Prazosin α₁
- Phentolamine

GENITO-URINARY SYSTEM: (see also "Urinary system"—p. 79)
aphrodisiac: yohimbe (relatively low dose & avoid other vasoconstricting meds and MAO-I)(H:D; 301); androstenedione (on theoretical grounds this may be effective; risks of concern-- see p. 48)
benign prostatic hypertrophy: saw palmetto (H:B+; 83, 406); several other herbs are of speculative value, including pumpkin seeds (H:D+; 406).
impotence: ginkgo (H:D; 300); yohimbe (H:D; 300)
infertility: alpinia (A:D; 83)
recurrent UTI's: cranberry and blueberry (H:B, 391, 221).
Recurrent yeast infections: oral echinacea after treating with topical antifungal cream (H:B; 316).

GYNECOLOGY (See also OBSTETRICS)
- **contraceptive activity:** blue cohosh (A:C; 83); gotu kola (A:D; 83); neem oil (1 ml intravag.)(L:B; H:D; 83)
- **dysmenorrhea:** black cohosh (A:C; 301); dong quai (H:C; 301); peppermint (H:B; 301)
- **fibrocystic breast changes:** primrose oil (H:D; 83; 301)
- **infertility:** to lengthen luteal phase—chaste tree (H:C; 83); flax seeds (H:D; 83)
- **menopause:** mainly for symptoms of estrogen withdrawal—black cohosh (H:C; 83, 301, 406); soybeans (H:C+; 317). The following herbs and foods have at least some supportive data, and are described in detail by Soffa (278): dong quai, black haw, chaste tree, fenugreek, hops, liferoot, pomegranate, red clover, wild yam, sage, hawthorn, sweet briar, raspberry, strawberry, and patented formulations of Chinese Herbs (H:C-D; 278).
- **post-operation stress:** ginseng (H:C-; 83); music (H:C;109).
- **PMS:** correct nutritional imbalances when present (H:B; 317); calcium supplementation (1200 mg elemental calcium, as calcium carbonate, every day) (H:B; 470); chaste tree (H:C-; 83, 374); dong quai (H:D; 301, 374); ginkgo (vs breast engorgement)(H:C; 83); black cohosh (A:C; 83); primrose (H:D; 301 & 83); Vitex (H:D)
- **smooth muscle relaxant:** raspberry (tea)(H:D; 301)
- **uterine contraction stimulant (emmenagogue):** blue cohosh (H:C; 83)
- **vaginitis:** echinacea (PO in combination with topical econazole vag. Cream greatly reduced the recurrence rate of vaginal candidiasis) (H:B; 316); yogurt in water as douche (H:C-; 83)

IMMUNE SYSTEM:

- **vs allergies:** perilla (A:C; 83); desensitization shots (orthodoxy)
- **vs age related decline in immune function:**
1. good nutrition (consider dietitian's review/supplement if deficient)(H:B; 20, 45, 46); screen for the following in geriatric females: protein calorie malnutrition, - cholesterol and DM (H:A; 198).
2. moderate endurance-type exercise (H:B; 213, 270)
- **factors that decrease immunity:** stress (H:B; 152); depression (H:C; 16); lack of sleep (H:C; 543).
- **factors that increase or improve immunity:** optimum nutrition (best evidence for such nutrition coming from food; specific dietary assessment and directed supplementation where indicated also with proven value—e.g., in zinc deficiency) (H:A; 45, 46; 198); light to moderate exercise (H:B-; 228; 268); biofeedback & other "mind-body" self regulation training (H:B-; 116); sufficient sleep (H:C; 543); basketball training & playing (note: transient decline in immunity with exhaustive activity)(H:C-; 21); echinacea (H:C; 83); eleutherococcus (H:C-; 83); cat's claw (L:B; 83).

INFECTIOUS DISEASE

ANTIBACTERIAL: (SEE ALSO SPECIFIC DISEASE OR SYNDROME, SUCH AS UTI) goldenseal, barberry and Oregon grape root all contain berberine which has antibacterial effects (H:B; 316); cranberry (decreases bacterial adherence)(H:B; 301, 316); garlic (L:B; H:B; 83, 301); xylitol (vs. Strep pneumonia as cause of otitis media)(H:B; 304); pineapple stem extract (bromelain)(H:C; 316); apple (extracts from bark, leaves & root- phloretin)(L:B; 83);burdock (fresh roots)(L:D; 301); calendula (L:D+; 83); cumin (L:C; 83); lemon verbena (L:C; 83); mace (L:C; 83); neem (CI- in small children)(L:D+; 83); propolis (L:C; H:C-; 301, 83); St. John's wort (L:C; 83); savory (L:C; 83); storax (H:D; 83); taheebo (L:C-; 83); woodruff (H:D; 83); acupuncture (A:C; 534).

ANTIFUNGAL: echinacea (to prevent recurrence of vaginal candidiasis)(H:B; 316); garlic (L:B; H:C; 83, 316); alpinia (L:B; 83); goldenseal, barberry and Oregon grape root all contain berberine which may have antifungal effects (L:C; 316); burdock (fresh roots)(L:D; 301); celery (oil)(L:C; 83); cinnamon (L:C-; 83); clove (esp. oil)(H:C; 83); melaluca oil (topical) (H:C; 83); mace (L:C; 83); propolis (L:C; H:C-; 301; 83); savory (L:C; 83); taheebo (L:C-; 83); trillium (L:C; 83)

ANTIMICROBIAL (MIXED OR UNSPECIFIED): barberry (bacteria & protozoa)(H:D; 301); bayberry (L:D; 301); burdock (A:C-; 83); chamomile (H:C; 301); eleutherococcus (L:C-; 83); fenugreek (bacteria & fungi)(A:C; 301); hibiscus (L:C; A:C; 83); myrrh (L:C; 83); royal jelly (L:D+; 83); sage (L:C; 83)

ANTIVIRAL (SEE ALSO SPECIFIC VIRUS OR DISEASE): asparagus (L:C; 83); calendula (L:C-; 83); propolis (L:C-; 83); St. John's wort (A:D+; 83)
- **common cold:** avoid exhaustive exercise (H:A; 214, 215); echinacea (H:B-; 258, 301, 410); zinc lozenges (H:C; 317); avoid or deal well with stresses (A:B;H:B; 152 ; 389); keep a variety of social ties (H:C+; 387); light exercise (H:C; 213-215); vitamin C supplements (slight effect only; H:C-; 390); remember the "orthodox" symptomatic treatments—mucolytics such as guaifenesin, decongestants such as pseudoephedrine, etc.
- **CMV:** yucca (L:C-; 83)
- **encephalitis:** tansy (vs tick borne enceph.) (narrow therapeutic window)(A:C-; 83); lentinan (intranasal, for prophylaxis; A:C-; 83)
- **hepatitis:** milk thistle extract (H:B-; 83, 301); aloe (PO or IV)(A:C; 83); ganoderma (vs. Hepatitis B: 171)(see also under GI—hepato-protective)
- **herpes:** capsicum peppers (vs post herpetic neuralgia—topical)(H:B; 83); cascara (L:C; 83); honey (H:D; 83); slippery elm (H:D; 83); yucca (L:C-; 83)
- **HIV:** burdock (L:C; 83); cat's claw (H:D; 83); hyssop (leaf extracts)(L:C; 83); St. John's wort (H:D; 83)
- **influenza:** avoid exhaustive exercise (H:A; 213-215); echinacea (H:C-; 35); garlic (L:C; 316)
- **polio:** grape juice (H:C-; 83)
- **rotavirus:** (gastroenteritis): valerian (H:C; 316)

ANTI-PARASITIC:
- **vs amoeba:** berberine (from goldenseal, barberry or Oregon grape root)(L:C; 316)
- **anti-helminthic** (vs worms): allspice (L:C; 83); cucurbita (pumpkin seeds)(H:C; 301; 83); cumin (L:C)
- **bilharzia-induced bladder lesions:** gotu kola (IM extracts)(H:C+; 83)
- **vs giardia:** berberine (from goldenseal, barberry or Oregon grape root)(H:C; 316)
- **vs leishmaniasis:** berberine (L:C; 316)
- **malaria:** quinine (cinchona bark extract)(H:A; 83); Artemisia species (H:C to D; 69, 372); gelsemium (H:D?; 69); neem (oil extracts)(CI- small children)(L:C-; 83)
- **schistosomiasis:** ginger (H:C; 372); tonka bean (H:D-; 83)

- **vs trypanosomes:** taheebo (L:C-; 83)

VS. ECTOPARASITES:
- fleas: tea tree (H:C-; 301)
- scabies: turmeric + neem (topical) (H:B-; 83)
- lice— manual removal and hygiene or call national pediculosis association (617)449-NITS or check their website: www.headlice.org

TOPICAL ANTISEPTICS: allspice (L:C; 83); tea tree (H:C; 301 & 83); tolu balsam (H:C-; 83)

URINARY TRACT INFECTION (UTI): cranberry juice (1 glass of 6-8 ounces BID probably sufficient for main therapeutic effect—inhibits bacterial adhesion)(H:B+; 301, 391); uva ursi (requires alkaline urine)(H:C+; 83 & 301); buchu (H:C; 301).

GASTROENTERITIS (GE): agrimony (H:B; 83, 406); goldenseal (berberine is active ingredient & is sold separately)(H:B; 316); savory (H:C-; 301)

YEAST INFECTIONS: echinacea (when given PO in combination with topical econazole, greatly decreased recurrence rates of vaginal candidiasis)(H:B; 316)

PHARYNGITIS: (remember penicillin is "natural" and prevents rheumatic heart disease): echinacea (immune stimulating effect)(H:B; 316); goldenseal (for berberine extract)(H:B; 316); vitamin C (weak positive effect)(H:C; 317); zinc lozenges (modest inhibition of viral replication in mucosa)(H:C-; 317). The following may give symptomatic relief: marsh mallow root (H:C; 301); slippery elm bark (H:C; 301); savory (H:C-; 83)

TUBERCULOSIS: adequate nutrition (H:B; 45, 46, 393); sunshine (or UV light)-decreases number of airborne infective organisms (L:A; 392); propolis (H:C-; 83; 301)

LONGEVITY
- **lifestyle: 7 health habits associated with longevity:** never smoke, moderate use of alcohol, daily breakfast, no snacking, 7-8 hours of sleep/night, regular exercise and maintain ideal weight (5 or more of these habits has significant effect epidemiologically; presence of 7 habits has strong effect)(H:B+; 78). See "Lifestyle" p. 29 to 31.
- **honor your father and mother:** giving such honor to one's elders is associated with health and longevity in the traditional teachings of traditional African healers, Buddhism, Christianity, and Judaism. (see under "Spirituality"—p. 75).

- **Avoid osteoporotic fractures:** adequate calcium plus vitamin D intake, along with moderate weight-bearing exercise (and possible hormonal replacement—usual care). See table of nutrients, p.112.
- **Maintain social ties:** those who do, tend to live longer. (H:B+; 352-7).
- **Memory support:** active use plus consider use of ginkgo biloba and/or phosphatidylserine (see under neurology for references).

NERVOUS SYSTEM:
Alzheimer's dz: music tx (palliative)(H:C-; 3); phosphatidylserine (see under dementia below); ginkgo biloba (see dementia)
aphasia: melodic intonation tx (H:C; 19)
dementia: art tx (H:C; 177, 285); phosphatidylserine (100 mg orally TID improved memory)(H:B+; 516, 517, 518); ginkgo (H:C; 83); music tx (H:C; 243); alpinia (A:C; 83);
general: exercise improves CNS function (H:A-; 310)
diabetic neuropathy: primrose oil (H:C; 83)
insomnia: valerian (H:B; 372)
post herpetic neuralgia ("shingles"): capsicum peppers (H:B; 394)
memory enhancement: to treat age-related memory decline: phosphatidylserine (H:B+; 516, 517, 518); ginkgo biloba (H:C; 83); to recall facts learned in the presence of an aroma, have the same aroma present when tested (H:C?; 599).
migraine: feverfew (esp. to prevent HA)(H:B; 83 & 301); (for recent review of orthodox & alternative tx, see Lewis, (170); acupuncture (H:C; 52); magnesium (from 200 mg Mg to 2 g MgSO4 per day; H:C; 316); yucca (H:D; 83)
multiple sclerosis: remember the recent advances in orthodox medicine, which has far better data than anything else we found; bee pollen or venom (not advised)(H:D; 83); weak electromagnetic fields (in picotesla range)(H:D; 255); light tx (H:D; 56); evening primrose oil(H:D; 83 & 301)
sedatives: kava kava (H:B+; 83); valerian (H:B; 372); chicory (H:C; 83 & 301); gotu kola (H:C; 301); hawthorn (H:C?; 301); hops (H:C?; 301); passion flower (H:C; 301)
seizures (epilepsy): ketogenic diet (starts with 1 to 3 day fast)(H:B; 6, 73); barberry (H:D; 301); celery (extract)(A:C; 83).
stimulants: caffeine (coffee, guarana, kola, mate', green tea)(H:A; 83 & 301); ephedra (H:A; 301); exercise (1 to 6 hour effect following moderately vigorous exercise)(H:B; 395)
stroke: most relevant risk factors: smoking, lack of exercise, high cholesterol and HTN.

Stroke rehabilitation: music tx (H:B-; 240); acupuncture (H:C; 234).

OBSTETRICS
- **orthodoxy** (midwifery or GP/Family practice with surgical or obstetric specialist availability; protocols modified by research, case reviews and panel conferences)(H:B+; 396, 398).
- **antimutagens:** asparagus (high in folic acid)(L:B; 83); eleutherococcus (A:C-; 83)
- **vs. nausea and vomiting** of pregnancy: acupressure, ginger and vitamin B6 supplementation all have fair supporting data for efficacy, though the acupressure data was at times contradictory. (H:C; 567).
- **prevention of obstetrical complication or need of C/S:** presence of a doula (H:B; 397)
- **pain control:** Lamaze method, (and other mind-body pain control methods)(H:B; 398); acupuncture (H:B; 528, 530); acupuncture also decreased time in labor (H:C; 528).
- **pregnancy induced hypertension:** may be prevented by adequate intake of linoleic acid and calcium (H:B; 539)—efficacy was shown using daily supplements of 450 mg of linoleic acid and 600 mg of calcium; qigong (essentially tai chi chuan) may serve as a complementary therapy (H:C; 477)
- **prevention of obstetrical complications:** presence of doula (H:B; 397); homeopathy (H:C-; 131)
- **vs post partum perineal pain:** lavender oil in bath (H:C-; 83)

OPHTHALMOLOGY
- **Blindness:** art (tactile) therapy—palliative (H:C; 94)
- **Cataracts:** prevention—sunglasses which block UV (orthodox); antioxidant-containing foods (H:C) or supplements – esp. Vit A, B1,2,3 Vit C and E (H:C-; 181); honey (H:D-; 83);
- **Diabetic retinopathy:** bilberry (H:C-; 316); grape seed extract (H:D; 316)
- **Glaucoma:** pilocarpus (source of pilocarpine)(H:A; 406); coleus forskohlii (H:C+; 316); salvia miltiorrhiza (H:C; 316); marijuana (H:D+; 406)
- **vs Herpes of cornea:** honey (H:D; 83)
- **vs Macular degeneration**: diet optimized for antioxidant intake, and for intake of copper and zinc (H:B-C; 317); bilberry (H:C-; 316); ginkgo biloba (H:C; 316); taurine supplements (A:D; 317)
- **Night vision enhancement:** bilberry (H:C-; 83)
- **vs Retinitis pigmentosa:** bilberry (H:C-; 316).

PSYCHOLOGY: addictions: social and spiritual approaches (for example, Alcoholics Anonymous)(H:B?; 407, et al); acupuncture (alone:

H:D; combined with whole art of Chinese Medicine: H:C; 399); yoga (H:C; 448); schisandra (A:C; 301); optimum health diet (see p. 38).
- **adolescent psychological problems:** art therapy (H:C-; 274, 312); tai chi (currently under investigation?)
- **agitation, nervousness:** valerian (H:B; 301); biofeedback (H:A; 84, 95, 166); music (H:C; 49, 117, 251, 321)
- **anxiety:** (including unexplained anxiety and situational—such as perioperative): music (H:B; 49, 117, 251, 321); biofeedback (H:B+; 84; 95; 166); kava kava (H:B; 83); tai chi chuan (H:C; 474); acupuncture (A:C; 529).
- **aphrodisiac:** optimize lifestyle (to promote good general health) (see lifestyle); yohimbe (rel. low dose and must avoid other vasoconstrictor agents or MAO-I meds)(H:D)
- **attention deficit hyperactivity disorder:** diet modification still controversial—perhaps most often a placebo benefit, though some individuals have relevant food sensitivities. Individuals with atopic dermatitis more likely to benefit from an elimination diet. Tartrazine dye seems to affect some. Aspartame does not affect most. (H:B to C; 31, 250, 322); Feingold diet apparently shown to be merely a placebo effect for most individuals (H:A; 157); EEG biofeedback (H:B; 174); combination of behavior therapy, parent education and neurobiofeedback (H:B; 291); tai chi (currently under investigation?)
- **depression:** For an overview see ref. (132); light therapy (esp. if seasonal affective disorder)(H:A; 59; Solar Lite: 1-800-864-3883); exercise (H:B; 395); St. John's wort (H:B-; 83 & 301); acupuncture (H:C; 536); consider or screen for nutritional deficiency and treat when appropriate (should be usual care but often forgotten. Deficiencies of these may cause depression: thiamine, niacin, pyridoxine, folate, vitamin B-12 and vitamin C); music therapy (H:C; 117); spiritual approaches— see under "Spirituality"; ginseng (H:D; 301); magnetic brain stimulation (low doses)(H:D; 339).
- **empathy development:** art therapy (H:C-; 229)
- **general sense of well-being:** exercise (H:B; 310); appropriate participation in religion (H:C; 205); avoid or manage stress well (H:B; 152)
- **grief:** art therapy (H:C-; 260)
- **insomnia:** valerian (onset of action = 1 hour)(H:B; 83).
- **post-traumatic stress disorder:** art therapy (H:C-; 107)
- **sedative:** valerian (H:B; 83); kava kava (H:B; 83); barberry (H:D; 301).
- **schizophrenia:** art therapy (palliative)(H:C-; 302); music (palliative)(H:C; 293);

stress: combination of exercise, relaxation or "self regulation" techniques, including meditation and biofeedback (H:B+; 84,

95, 166, 407); kava kava (H:B; 83); ginseng (A:B; 83); optimize lifestyle habits (see under lifestyle); tai chi chuan (H:C; 474).

RESPIRATORY SYSTEM: (see also ENT)

- **asthma:** ephedra (has stimulant—beta-mimetic effects)(H:A; 301); ammi (requires careful monitoring for eye & liver toxicity)(H:B; 83); optimized dietary vitamin C intake (H:B; 120; 261); massage (H:B; 401); yoga and breathing techniques (H:C; 450); coltsfoot (L:B; H:D; 83).
- **bronchitis & congestion:** myrrh (decongestant action)(H:C; 301)
- **demulcent** (soothes mucous membranes): licorice (H:A; 301); tragacanth (H:C-; 83).
- **vs desaturations in neonates:** massage (H:B; 401); music (H:C; 282).
- **expectorants:** senega snakeroot (H:B; 301); horehound (H:C+; 83 & 301); hyssop (H:D; 83 & 301); licorice (H:A; 301); squill (narrow therapeutic window)(H:C+; 83); tolu balsam (H:C-; 83); yerba santa (H:D; 83)
- **mechanical ventilation :** for review on how to treat patient distress at being on ventilator, see Fontaine (87).

RHEUMATOLOGY:
analgesia (versus pain)—topical (external use only): wintergreen oil (H:C; 83)
anti-inflammatory: juniper (H:C-; 83); propolis (A:C; 83)
verses arthritis (in general): acupuncture (H:B for osteoarthritis; less data for other types; 209); aloe (topical)(H:D; 83); alpinia (A:D; 83); bee venom (A:B; H:D; risks include anaphylaxis and with multiple stings: renal failure; 83); Ben Gay® (H:C-; 209); capsaicin (H:C- for osteoarthritis; less data for other types; 209); chamomile (A:C-; 83); compression gloves (H:C; 209); copper bracelets (H:D; 209); devil's claw (A:C; 83); feverfew (H:C+, esp. prophylactic; 83; 301); glucosamine (H:B+; 83); heat & cold topical treatments (H:C-; 209); spa therapy (heat, rest, exercise)(H:D; 209); TENS (H:B- for osteoarthritis and rheumatoid arthritis; H:C for ankylosing spondylitis; 209); turmeric (A:C-; 83); yucca (H:D; 83, 301)
vs carpal tunnel syndrome: yoga (H:C; 465)
connective tissue protectant: pycnogenol (A:C; 83)
vs. Fibromyalgia: acupuncture (H:C; 271); for comparison of conventional and alternative treatments see the review by Simms (271).
Vs Lupus: flax seeds (A:D; 83); UV- A1 phototherapy (H:C-; 55); DHEA supplementation (H:C; 558). See page 49 for discussion of safety concerns with DHEA.

vs Osteoarthritis: (see also vs. Arthritis): glucosamine (H:B+; 83)
vs post-traumatic arthritis: (see also vs. Arthritis): glucosamine (H:B; 83)
vs rheumatoid arthritis: (see also vs. Arthritis): tai chi chuan (as a suitable exercise therapy) (H:C; 475); primrose oil (H:C-; 83)

SPIRITUALITY: In recent times we have followed the dictum, "In God we trust. All others must present data." However, for that insatiable desire to learn more, we seek to discover the data that does exist linking some aspects of spirituality to health.

Good reviews of relevant data have been published by Benson (407) and by Daniel P. Wirth (461, 462). Both authors document the powerful effect of faith on healing. Such faith seems to be effective when sincere on the part of the patient – independent of the patient's particular religious persuasion (H:A; 407). (Even agnostics benefited when they had faith in something, someone or some cause). Other spiritual principles demonstrated to be effective include meditation (H:A; 407), participation in ceremonies, belonging to a supportive group, and participating in altruistic deeds, (approx. H:B; 407, 461, 462). There is good data that prayer works when the patient is aware that it is taking place. (H:B+; 407, 408). Prayer done when the patient is unaware of such support has positive data from one good study involving almost 400 patients—but this study has some valid potential sources of error and has apparently not be reproduced. (408).

Historical insights into spirituality's role in healing, along with examples of how some physicians try to re-introduce the spiritual side of healing, are nicely presented in Daniel Wirth's 1993 review, "Implementing Spiritual Healing in Modern Medical Practice."(462). Consensus on how to integrate spirituality with modern medicine seems beyond reach. However, we all, as health professionals would do well to foster the faith and sense of meaning among our patients.

Students of spirituality and of religion well know that faith can also harm when it is mis-directed. To this end the neglect of providing basic and emergency medical care to children results in many preventable deaths, as was recently documented in a review in the journal Pediatrics (H:B+; 454). In the review, authors Rita Swan PhD and Seth Asser MD reviewed 172 deaths among children whose families depended upon faith healing to the exclusion of usual care. They found that 81% of the deaths were caused by conditions that had a 90% or greater chance of survival had usual care been rendered. This prompted Dr. Swan to observe, "This is Jonestown in slow motion!"—a chilling reference to the editors of this little book as most of us live near where many of the victims of the Jonestown incident lived. Twenty years ago, 900 followers of Rev. Jim Jones joined him in a bizarre mass suicide. (455, 456).

Following are some **observations from some major world religions:**

Thus far the editors have collected relevant teachings from Buddhism, African traditional healers, and from Judeo-Christian teachings. (We welcome relevant input regarding other religions' health teachings). For much of world history, and still to some degree today, the roles of physician and priest are the same. In the above belief systems, as well as in Islam and in Hinduism, one's peace with Divinity is important to health. Various moral absolutes have also been included. Interestingly, one of the more common of these we have found so far is the directive to honor one's parents (or elders).

African traditional religions: health and illness are often viewed as being under the major influence of social relations. Family, tribe and ancestors (sometimes viewed as deified) affect one's health. Respect for elders (and ancestors) is important. Healing may depend upon correcting a strained relationship involving the spiritual, psychological and social context of the patient. (478). Medicinal herbs are often prescribed.

Buddhism: As in most great religions, faith and morality are the foundation of the religion. Five basic moral directives are held They are:

1) Do not kill. (This may include a tendency to avoid fighting and war. Such avoidance may save many from an untimely demise. Some schools of Buddhism also include in this moral principle the teaching to be vegetarian—which is associated with many health benefits—see. p. 42).
2) Do not steal.
3) Do not engage in sexual misconduct. (Obeyed, this avoids serious and potentially life-threatening infections as well as various social problems).
4) Do not speak falsely.
5) Do not take intoxicants. (This means abstaining from alcohol, tobacco and various "recreational" drugs. Such abstinence prevents much disability and premature death).

In addition, honoring elders is taught to be associated with improving health and improving one's life span. Further, abandoning anger and pride are associated with improved health (442).

Buddhism does not shun modern healers, in fact, their tradition is to respect them and honor their efforts. Buddhist custom and belief should be consulted, however, so as to not make the patient or their family unduly uncomfortable. (One Buddhist teaching that may require some advance consideration is that a body should not be moved for the first eight hours after death, so as to "not disturb the spirit.")

Traditional thought in Buddhism teaches that illness may be the result of deterioration of the body (as in aging) or the result of "bad karma," (in one's present or previous life). As a local Buddhist monk, Heng Shun, explains,

"..."Karma" literally means "activity." Karma (in Buddhism) is specifically the activities we do over and over again—activities rooted in desire and governed by the law of cause and effect. The law of cause and effect, simply stated, is that every good or bad act of body, speech and thought, generates a corresponding good or bad result. The cause necessarily brings the result, which differs only in degree and time according to circumstances. This does not in anyway negate any scientific theories for the causes of illness, rather it indicates that behind these phenomena there is karma and the results of karma.

"If an illness is not a part of the natural process of aging, but rather a result of some karma in the past, there are several ways according to Buddhism, in which a person can counteract it (in addition to using medical techniques). The four most common methods found in the Buddhist Sutras (Sacred Texts) are reciting certain Sutras (in the Thervada tradition these texts are specifically called Parittas), reciting the holy names of Buddhas or Bodhisattvas (highly evolved spiritual beings, close to being Buddhas), reciting the names of mantras (spiritual words of great power taught by the Buddhas and Bodhisattvas), or doing good deeds with the intent to specifically counteract the illness. In all of these situations, the idea is to create new exceedingly good karma to go against the result of the bad karma that had been created in the past. Whether or not this will be successful depends on how great the force of the unwholesome karmic result is, and how strong one's spiritual or wholesome practices are. "

Judeo-Christian teachings on health also combine faith, morals, and good deeds. Further, public hygiene may have been introduced to at least a large part of the world from the Jews, since the time of the Exodus. With references to scriptural texts, here are some relevant teachings in various areas of health:

- general healing effects: love (H:B; 112); confession (Psalm 32:3); prayer (see above discussion) (H:B; 168, 407, 408); helping the poor and needy (Isa 58); honor and trust God, giving credit to God and turning away from evil (Prov. 3:3-8); Sabbath (Isa 58); joy (merry)(Prov 17:22); wise words spoken in a timely manner (as opposed to speaking rashly)(Prov 12:18); cheerful eye contact & good news (Prov 15:30); healing (at least eventual, incl. eternal life free from illness) by faith in God, knowing God, belief in the Son of God (John 3:16; 17:3; Rev 22:2; Psalm 103:3; Prov 3:3-8)
- Judeo-Christian examples of the integration of faith in God, forgiveness, and healing: Psalm 103:3; Prov 3:3-8; Luke 5:17-24; eventual restoration: cf. Gen 3:22-24 & Rev. 22:2.
- Longevity: honor your father and mother (one of the ten commandments—see Exodus 20).
- perspective: get your soul "right with God" and all other needs cared for (Ex. 20:1; Matt. 6:33); the kingdom of heaven is about righteousness, joy and peace, (not necessarily the immediate material and health blessings we want)- see Rom 14:17.
- empathy development: participation in art (H:D+; 229)
- Creator's design: seeks to understand the Creator's design for optimal lifestyle choices, and, insofar as practical, make changes in that direction. Examples include the aspects noted above, plus, where feasible, a vegetarian diet, exercise, hygiene, time allotted for prayer, meditation and rest, and other ideas variously held by individuals or groups. (Examples in Gen. 2, Daniel 1 & 2; see also under Lifestyles, p. 6)

Hinduism: moral considerations, healthy habits, use of meditation, prayer, yoga and herbs are all part of healing from a Hindu perspective. To some degree, Hinduism has borrowed from and absorbed Buddhism. (443, 444).

Islam: abstaining from alcohol and tobacco are advised, with obvious health benefits. Moral behavior, faith, and social support are also part of Islam and have positive health effects.

In contrast to Buddhism, bodies are to be washed, draped and prepared for burial as soon after death as is feasible.(445)

The observed month of daytime fasting, Ramadan, may affect health.(446) Depending upon quantity and quality of food eaten after sundown and before sunrise, this month of fasting may result in either fat gain or loss. Those living and working in hot, humid environments are at risk for dehydration during the day. Pregnant persons and those with illnesses are advised to postpone their observation of Ramadan until a more appropriate time. Illnesses that may place one at particular risk are peptic ulcer disease, heart and blood pressure conditions, hyperlipidemias, gout, and liver and kidney diseases. Observance of Ramadan may improve cellular immunity. (446).

TRAUMA & SURGERY:

- **anti-inflammatory & analgesic:** angelica topically (avoid PO) (L:B; A:B; 83)
- **anxiety pre- and post- op:** music (H:B; 49, 117, 321)
- **bone problems:** calm mind (H:B to C; 407, cf. in the Bible, Proverb 14:30); help the needy, call for Divine help and refrain from accusing others (H:C; 407, cf. in writings of Isaiah 58:6-11).
- **burns:** aloe (topical)(H:C-; 83); honey (topical)(H:C; 83)
- **frostbite:** aloe (H:C-; 83)
- **hemostasis** (stop bleeding): alchemilla (topical- skin)(H:C; 83); trillium (topical)(H:D+; 83); witch hazel (topical)(H:D+; 83)
- **transplant related problems:** Coenzyme Q (vs organ ischemia)(A:C; 83)
- **topical wound healing effects:** remember the role of optimum nutrition (orthodox but often forgotten)(H:A; 317); sugar (topical)(H:A; 317); honey (H:A; 83); glycosamino-glycans (H:C+; 317); maggots (raised for this purpose—"surgical maggots")—for debridement (H:A; 83)—common side effect is itching!; arnica (H:C; 83 & 301); myrrh (H:C; 301); echinacea (A:B; 83); propolis (H:C-; 83); tea tree (H:C; 301); allspice (L:C; 83); calendula (A:C; 83, 301); gotu kola (A:B-; L:B-; 83); yarrow (H:C-; 83)woodruff (H:D; 83).
- **internal wound healing:** remember optimum nutrition (orthodoxy)(H:A; 317).

URINARY SYSTEM (UROLOGY)—(see also "genito-urinary system"):

- **anti-diuretic:** savory (H:C-; 83)
- **vs bladder spasms:** cat's claw (A:C; 83)

- **diuretics:** lovage (H:B; 301); mate' (H:B-; 83); nettle (H:B; 301); uva ursi (H:B; 83); artichoke (H:C; 83); boldo (A:A; H:B; 83); buchu (H:C; 83); burdock (A:C; 83); dandelion (A:A; 83); alpinia (A:C; 83); fenugreek (A:C-; 83); hibiscus (H:D?; 301); juniper (caution re: renal toxicity; avoid in pregnancy)(H:C-; 83 & 301).
- **infertility:** zinc deficiency is associated with infertility (male & female)(H:C; 71)
- **prostate cancer:** intake of tomato sauce is associated with decreased risk of prostate CA (H:B-; 429-430); eating garlic twice/week was associated with halving the risk of prostate CA (H:C; 439); deficiency of zinc is associated with increased risk of prostate CA (H:C; 71)
- **prostatitis:** zinc deficiency is associated with prostatitis (H:C-; 71)
- **prostatic enlargement** (Benign Prostatic Hypertrophy): BPH is associated with xs zinc (H:C; 71); pygeum extract (an herbal product) is safe and effective treatment for BPH (H:B; 83); cucurbita (pumpkin) seeds (H:D; 301); nettle (H:D; 301); saw palmetto (fat soluble fraction is active—not water based teas)(H:B; 301, 406)
- **stones:** selected diets & increase water intake (orthodoxy); burdock (H:D; 83); fenugreek (A:C-; 83)— decreases renal calcium oxalate precipitation
- **urinary tract infection:** cranberry (H:B; 391)—6 to 8 ounces of juice twice a day is effective (prevents adherence of E. coli bacteria).

TABLE OF HERBS AND SELECTED FOODS

NAME	ACTIVITY	ADVERSE EFFECTS	GRAS*	EXAMPLE OF FORM AND DOSE**	REF.
acacia gum	vs irritated mucous memb. (H:C); prevents dental plaque (H:C)	occl severe allergies	yes	PO (up to 3 g TID); topical; chew	69, 83
acerola	excellent source of vitamin C	considered safe	no	PO (250 mg caps qd to TID)	83
acidophilus	vs antibiotic induced diarrhea (H:C); vs UTI (L:B; 307); vs campylobacter pylori (L:B; 23); may lower cholesterol and prevent some cancers (H:C; 194); to prevent candidal vaginitis	considered safe	n/a	PO	23, 76, 83, 194, 307.
aconite	none in safe doses	CV & CNS toxicity	no	not advised	83
agrimony	vs pharyngitis (symptomatic) (H:C-); vs diarrhea (H:C-)	photodermatitis	no	topical; PO (1-2 tsp. dried leaves used to make 1 cup tea TID)	69, 83
alchemilla	vs bleeding (topical)(H:C); antioxidant (H:C)	potential hepatotoxicity or carcinogen with chronic use	no	topical; PO	83
aletris	estrogenic (L:D)	uncertain	no	PO (0.5 g dried root)	83
alfalfa	none known	probably safe; (may worsen SLE?; reversible pancytopenia)	yes	PO (sprouts added as one would to a salad)	69, 83, 301, 316
allspice	antihelminth (L:C); antioxidant (L:C); topical antiseptic/anesthetic(H:D)	irritation of muc. mem.; xs oil → CNS & GI toxicity	yes	topical; PO (up to 2g daily)	69, 83

See KEY and important information on p. 17-19. Abbreviations are listed on p. 163. Doses given are examples only. Read product labels carefully!

*Generally recognized as safe by the FDA.
**Doses vary widely-- read labels carefully!

Table of Herbs and Selected Foods

HERB	ACTIVITY	RISKS	gras	EXAMPLE OF DOSE	REF.
aloe	anti-inflammatory (burns—incl. sunburn; frostbite)(H:C); anti-septic (L:C); vs arthritis (H:C-); vs hepatitis (A:C); laxative (very strong)(H:A)	dermatitis; GI cramps (PO); PO CI in pregnancy and children	yes	topical; PO (up to 30 ml/dose)	5, 83, 300, 301, 316
alpinia	see galangal				
ammi	↑'s HDL (khellin der. from ammi)(H:C); vs angina (H:B); vs asthma (H:B); vs vitiligo (H:C); vs psoriasis (H:C)	↑ LFT's; N/V; monitor for pigmentary retinopathy	no	PO, IV, topical	83, 316
angelica	see dong quai				
apple	antibacterial (bark, leaves and root extract of phloretin)(L:A); vs constipation or diarrhea (fruit)(H:C); antimutagenic effects (varied by clutivar—best for Granny Smith and Red Delicious, fair for Golden Delicious) (L:B; 547).	xs seeds toxic due to cyanide content	n/a	PO (1- 2 per day typical)	69, 83, 547
apricot	The kernels have been used for a variety of ills, from asthma to vaginitis— apparently due to cytotoxic effect of the cyanide content (narrow therapeutic window!). (H:D)	Ingestion of as few as 2 kernels has been fatal. (H:B). Wild strains more potent than cultured. Excess fruit may be harmful (H:D)			69, 83
arnica	topical wound healing (H:C-)	topical considered safe; PO may → CV, CNS or GI toxicity	no	topical (tincture from flowers)	9, 69, 83, 300, 301

See KEY and important information on p. 17-19. Abbreviations are listed on p. 163. Doses given are examples only. Read product labels carefully!

Table of Herbs and Selected Foods

HERB	ACTIVITY	RISKS	gras	EXAMPLE OF DOSE	REF.
artichoke	↓'s glucose (H:D+); diuretic (H:C); hepato-protective (H:D); stimulates bile (H:B); prevents cancers (L:B; 2)	considered safe.	yes	PO	2, 83, 316
asparagus	antimutagen (L:C); antiviral (L:C)	considered safe	no	PO	83
aspidium	purges worms from gut (H:A)	moderate to profound weakness (dose related)	no	PO	83
autumn crocus	extracts (colchicine, etc.): vs CA (H:D); vs hepatitis (H:D); vs gout (H:A)	GI toxicity (potent)	no	not advised	69, 83
avocado	vs dry skin (oil) (H:C); ↓'s LDL (H:B)	(seeds and leaves have some toxicity)	no	PO	83
barberry	antibacterial (vs cholera)(H:C); sedative, local anesth. and vs. seizures}(H:D); ↑'s uterine CTXs (H:D)	xs → ↓ BP; diarrhea; nephritis	no	PO (about 1 g bark TID or use standardized teas or extracts)	69, 83, 301, 316
barley	sympathomimetic (root)(H:B); ↓'s LDL (whole grain & oil)(H:C); ↓'s HDL (whole grain)(H:C); ⁻ risk colon CA (A:C; H:D)	considered safe; (root—unknown)	n/a	PO	83
bayberry	vs diarrhea (H:D+)	carcinogenic (A:C); GI upset (H:C)	no	top.; PO not adv. (Usu. Is 1 g TID or standardized extract or decoction)	69, 83, 301
bearberry	see uva ursi				
bee pollen	speculative & anecdotal—none with good evidence found	allergies, including anaphylaxis	n/a	PO	83

See KEY and important information on p. 17-19. Abbreviations are listed on p. 163. Doses given are examples only. Read product labels carefully!

HERB	ACTIVITY	RISKS	gras	EXAMPLE OF DOSE	REF.
bee venom	vs arthritis (A:B; H:D); desensitization shots (H:C); vs MS (H:D-	anaphylaxis; renal failure (with many stings)	n/a	SQ	83
bergamot	vs psoriasis & vitiligo (extracts)}H:D	photodermatitis (H:B); possible carcinogens (A:D)	yes	topical; PO	83
betel nut	cathartic (A:C); anti-helminth (A:C)	CV & CNS toxic (seeds); gingivitis, periodontal dz, oral leukoplakia and squamous cell CA (H:B+)	no	chewed (nut)	69, 83, 246
betony	cathartic/emetic (high doses)(H:D) vs diarrhea (mild-mod dose) (H:C); vs. nervous tension (H:C)	high in tannins; sl ↓ BP (H:D); avoid in pregnancy (theoretical embryotoxic effects of polyphenols)	no	PO	69, 83, 301
bilberry fruit	vs diarrhea (mild)(H:C); vs edema (A:C+); improves night vision (H:C-); vs pharyngitis (symptomatic)(H:C); vs PUD (A:C); protects vs xs vaso-permeability due to HTN	considered safe; (high doses and chronic use?-- contains tannins)	no	PO; topical; (animals-IV)	83, 316
Bioflavo-noids (myricetin, silymarin, quercetin, et al)	inhibits tumor growth (L:B; 70; A:B: 146); Silymarin vs complicated DM in cirrhotic patients (H:C+; 308); Silymarin vs cisplatin-induced renal toxicity (A:B; 29)	generally safe from foods, except concerns re: milk thistle (silymarin)—see milk thistle		PO, IV	29, 146, 308

See KEY and important information on p. 17-19. Abbreviations are listed on p. 163. Doses given are examples only. Read product labels carefully!

Table of Herbs and Selected Foods

HERB	ACTIVITY	RISKS	gras	EXAMPLE OF DOSE	REF.
black cohosh	vs menopausal sympt. (H:C)	↓'ed BP, GI upset, esp. with excessive doses	no	PO (typically taken as standardized extracts: 4 mg TID or as per label; decoction from 1 tsp. root TID or 1 ml tincture TID)	5, 69, 83, 300, 301, 316
bloodroot	vs dental plaque (H:A); vs skin CA (A:B; H:D+)	xs →CNS depression, N/V	no	topical; dental (decoction from 1 tsp. dried rhizome TID or tincture 1 ml TID)	69, 83, 316
blue cohosh	inhibits ovulation (A:C-); ↑'s uterine CTXs (H:C)	constricts coronary arteries (A:C)	no	PO (decoction from 1 tsp. dried root or 1 ml tincture TID)	69, 83, 301
blueberry	vs UTI (L:B; 221)	safe	n/a	PO	221
boldo	stimulates bile (H:B-); diuretic (H:B)	xs →CNS & musc. stimulation then depression/paralysis	yes	PO	69, 83
boneset	extracts may have research value (vs CA, clotting, & immunity)	xs → diarrhea (H:B); hepatotoxic with chronic use (H:C)	no	not advised	69, 83, 301
Boswellia serrata—see Frankincense					
brewer's yeast	↓'s LDL, ↑'s HDL and ↑'s glucose tolerance (H:B+); may improve acne (H:D+)	considered safe	n/a	20 g per day	317

See KEY and important information on p. 17-19. Abbreviations are listed on p. 163. Doses given are examples only. Read product labels carefully!

Table of Herbs and Selected Foods

HERB	ACTIVITY	RISKS	gras	EXAMPLE OF DOSE	REF.
broom	vs dysrhythmias (H:C)	CV, CNS toxicity and ↑ uterine CTXs	no	not advised	83, 301
buchu	diuretic (mild)(H:C); antibacterial (mild)(H:D)	considered safe	yes	PO (tea from 1 tsp. dried leaves or 1 ml tincture TID)	69, 83, 301
burdock	vs dandruff, fevers, HIV, microbes, renal stones}(L:C- H:D) mild diuretic (H:C)	considered safe; occl allergies; occl contamination	no	topical; PO (decoction from 1 tsp. dried root TID or 1 ml tincture TID)	69, 83, 301, 316
butcher's broom	anti-inflammatory (A:C); vs varicose vv (H:C-)	considered safe	no	PO	83, 300, 301, 316
cajeput	see melaleuca				
calabar bean	strong cholinergic	physostigmine related CV and Resp. effects		not advised	83
calamus	antispasmotic (sm. mm relaxant)(A:C); sedative (A:A)	possible source of carcinogens and mutagens	no	not advised	83, 301
calendula officinalis (pot marigold)	antibacterial & antiviral (L:C-); anti-inflammatory (A:C-); wound healing (A:C); vs periodontal dz (A:D); vs PUD (A:D); vs CA (A:C)	allergies (with one case of anaphylaxis reported)	yes	topical; PO (tea from 1 tsp. dried flowers or 1 ml tincture TID)	69, 83, 300, 301
canaigre	vs tumors (L:C-)	high in tannins (theor. risk carcinogenicity)	yes	top.; PO not adv.	69, 83, 301
capers	improves capillary integrity & vs dry skin (H:D+)	dermatitis	yes	topical	83
capsicum pepper	vs pain of shingles (H:B); other pains (H:C-); anticarcinogen (H:C-)	may ↑ pain (usu. temporary); very irritating to muc. mem. (H:B); carcinogenic? (H:C-)	yes	topical	69, 119, 289, 301, 316

See KEY and important information on p. 17-19. Abbreviations are listed on p. 163. Doses given are examples only. Read product labels carefully!

Table of Herbs and Selected Foods

HERB	ACTIVITY	RISKS	gras	EXAMPLE OF DOSE	REF.
cardamom	prevents aflatoxin-related cancer (L:B)	safe		PO	119
carob	vs. diarrhea (H:C)	occl allergies		PO	427
carrot oil	hepato-protective (A:C); vs HTN (Ca-channel blocker effect)(A: C)	considered safe; xs seeds or seed oil may → CNS toxicity	yes	PO (seed oil or root oil)	83
cascara	↓'s cholesterol (A:C); vs constipation (H:A); vs hepatoma (L:C); vs herpes (L:C); vs leukemia (A:C); sunscreen (H:C-)	CI- pregnancy, ileus. fresh—severe GI cramps/vomiting; chronic use → ↓ K, dependence; melanosis coli	yes	topical; PO (decoction from 1 tsp. dried bark or 1 ml tincture BID)	5, 69, 83
castor	laxative (oil) H:A	beans, leaves and seeds may be fatal taken internally (PO)		oil-PO	83, 316
cat's claw	vs bladder spasms (A:C); vs HIV (H:D); vs HTN (A:B); immune-enhancing (L:B); vs mutagens (L:C; H:D)	considered safe		PO	83
celery	vs CA (A:C); fungicidal (oil) (L:C); vs HTN (A:C); sedative (A:C); may lower cholesterol (A:C; 298); may prevent aflatoxin-related cancer (animal model using extracts from celery (L:C; 119)	CNS depression; diseased plants may contain carcinogens		PO (tea from 1 tsp. fresh seeds or 1 ml tincture TID); topical?	27; 69; 83; 298; 119
Centipeda minima	Effective vs. bacterial sinusitis (L:B; 568). (a traditional Nepalese herb)	unknown		PO	568

See KEY and important information on p. 17-19. Abbreviations are listed on p. 163. Doses given are examples only. Read product labels carefully!

Table of Herbs and Selected Foods

HERB	ACTIVITY	RISKS	gras	EXAMPLE OF DOSE	REF.
chamomile	anti-inflammatory (A:B); antispasmotic (GI) (H:C-D); vs arthritis (A:C-D); vs PUD (A:C); vs stress (A:B)	allergies, including anaphylaxis		PO	5, 69, 83, 316, 328
chaparral	vs CA (L:B; H:D)	hepato-toxicity; may worsen some cancers		PO (not adv)	83, 301, 316
charcoal	vs poisoning (H:A); vs xs gas (H:C)	xs→ GI obstruction (H:B); aspiration		PO (0.5 to 1 g/kg, max. 90 g, up to Q 4 Hr	83
chaste tree	vs PMS (H:C;); vs xs PRL-related menstrual irregularity (H:C-)	occasional GI upset or rash		PO (dried berries 1 tsp. in tea TID or tincture up to 20 mg per day)	5, 83
chestnut	see horse chestnut				
chicory	anti-inflammatory (A:C-D); sedative (H:C); quinidine-like effect slows heart rate (A:C-D)............	considered safe	yes	PO (60 g in 1 liter tea; div. TID)	83, 301
Chinese cucumber	Vs. HIV (L:B); vs. melanoma, hepatoma and other neoplasms (H:C)	May cause abortion; fairly narrow therapeutic window of extracts (multi-organ system adverse effects reported, esp. with unsupurvised IV use)			83

See KEY and important information on p. 17-19. Abbreviations are listed on p. 163. Doses given are examples only. Read product labels carefully!

Table of Herbs and Selected Foods

chocolate	pleasant effects on mood – perhaps due to stimulant effects of theobromine, caffeine and phenylethylamine (the latter speculated to produce feelings as if one is in love); increases serotonin release (H:C; 404, 435); antioxidant effects (L:B; 402, 403); mild effect vs asthma L:C)	headaches in small % of individuals (H:C-; 317); no apparent specific comedogenic properties (H:C-; 317); concern over role in fibrocystic breast dz seems unwarranted. (H:B; 428, 431, 432)	PO 20-90 g per "dose"	317; 402-4; 435
cinnamon	vs CHF (↑ ANF→diuresis) (A:C-D); vs diarrhea (A:C-); vs fungi (oral and respiratory)(L:B+; H:C-); prevents toxic histamine formation in fish (L:B; 264); vs bacteria (static)(L:B; 336); vs PUD (A:B; 292)	xs →vasomotor instability; dermatitis; oral leucoplakia; mucous membrane irritation (H:B; 231)	PO (0.5 to 1 g up to TID)	11, 69, 83, 241, 273
clematis	androgenic (A:D); anti-inflammatory (H:C-D); CNS stimulant (A:C); hepatoprotective (A:C-D); vs HTN (A:C-D); skin disorders (H:D)	skin irritation; potentially serious GI or renal toxicity	topical; PO not advised	69, 83

See KEY and important information on p. 17-19. Abbreviations are listed on p. 163. Doses given are examples only. Read product labels carefully!

HERB	ACTIVITY	RISKS	gras	EXAMPLE OF DOSE	REF.
clove	vs dermatophytosis (H:C); vs toothache (H:A); vs "dry socket" (H:A); vs PUD (A:C-D); vs CA (A:C-D); spasmolytic (H:D); prevents toxic histamine formation in fish (L:B; 264); inhibits platelet aggregation (oil extract) (L:B).	considered safe, (unless smoked which occasionally → severe pulmonary toxicity)	gras	PO/ oral mucosa; topical (esp. the oil)	69, 83; 264
cocoa	see chocolate				
coenzyme Q	ergogenic (H:D-); vs ischemic heart dz (A:C); vs. CHF (H:C); vs. transplant-related ischemia (A:B); vs. drug or toxin related hepatoxicity and rhabdomyolysis (eg. Due to lovastatin and carbon tetrachloride) (A:B; H:D).	considered safe; (unknown in pregnancy)	n/a	PO	83, 436, 437
coffee	stimulant & diuretic (H:A); may inhibit gallstone formation	palpitations; insomnia; GERD; xs (5 cups or more/d ?):↑ risk atherosclerosis in men (H:C); - gallbladder CTX		PO (1 to 4 cups as infusion, per day)	317, 405
cola acuminata	This is the common "cola" used in soft drinks, and contains avg. 1.8% caffeine and about 0.1% (max) theobromine. CNS stimulant and beta-mimetic effects (H:A, 69); vs. viral infections (L:B)	Theoretical risk of cancer and teratogenicity though data in animals and humans is sparse.		PO	69

See KEY and important information on p. 17-19. Abbreviations are listed on p. 163. Doses given are examples only. Read product labels carefully!

Table of Herbs and Selected Foods

HERB	ACTIVITY	RISKS	gras	EXAMPLE OF DOSE	REF.
cola nitida	Sometimes used in cola drinks and chewed traditionally; contains avg. 3% caffeine and 1% theobromine. Effects as for cola acuminata—may be effective vs. diarhea.	As for cola acuminata.		PO	69
coltsfoot	vs asthma (L:B; H:D); vs pain of sore throat (H:B)	with chronic use may have significant amt. carcinogen		PO (dried flowers: 1 tsp. in infusion or 3 ml tincture TID)	69
comfrey	anti-inflammatory (topical) (A:C-D)	contains pyrrolizidine alkaloids—xs or chronic use may → hepatic dz or be carcinogenic		caution advised (1 tsp. dried root or leaves as decoction or tea up to TID)	300, 301
cordyceps sinensis	vs. Leukemic cells (L:B; 48); immunosuppressive activity (L:B; 161); to protect vs. Aminoglycoside nephrotoxicity (H:C; 12); tumor growth inhibition (L:B; 162); vs lung CA (H:C); vs melanoma (A:C)	considered safe, though two cases of lead poisoning from contaminated cordyceps reported (H:C; 327)	no	PO	48, 369
coriander	prevents aflatoxin-related cancer (L:B)	safe		PO (up to 1 g TID)	119
cranberry	vs UTI (↓'es bacterial adherence with 6 oz PO BID) (H:B)	considered safe; GI upset with xs.		PO (180 ml juice BID)	301, 316;
cucumber, Chinese	vs DM (H:C-D); vs HIV (L:C)	cerebral and pulm. edema; seizures. (CI: pregnancy)		PO&IV: research protocols.	83

See KEY and important information on p. 17-19. Abbreviations are listed on p. 163. Doses given are examples only. Read product labels carefully!

Table of Herbs and Selected Foods

HERB	ACTIVITY	RISKS	gras	EXAMPLE OF DOSE	REF.
cumin	antibacterial (L:C); antihelminthic (L:C); anti-oxidant (A:C-D); may prevent aflatoxin-related cancers (L:B; 119); platelet inhibition (L:B; 288)	considered safe; recent case report of anaphylaxis (33)		PO (up to 1 g TID)	83; 119
damiana	aphrodisiac (H:0)	considered safe		PO (up to 300 mg dried leaves & stems TID)	83, 301
dandelion	vs DM (A:C); diuretic (A:A); vs irritable bowel syndrome (H:D)	considered safe (may cause drowsiness)		PO (leaves—30 to 90 g up to QID)	69, 83, 301
devil's claw	vs arthritis (A:C); vs cardiac arrhythmias (A:C-D); vs HTN (A:B)	rarely ↓ appetite; HA; tinnitus; long-term-?		PO (up to 500 mg TID)	69, 83, 301, 316
devil's club	vs DM (A:D-)	nausea, vomiting.	no	PO	83
devil's dung	none useful	methemoglobinemia in infants (L:C; H:D)	no	PO	83
digitalis	vs CHF (H:A-B); dysrhythmias (H:A)	narrow therapeutic window, fatal in xs.	no	R'x. pills PO	69, 83, 316
dolomite	calcium and magnesium source	occl. heavy metal contamination	no	PO	83
dong quai	vs allergies (A:C); CNS stimulant (A:C); vs dysmenorrhea (H:D); vs menopausal sympt. (H:C); immune suppressant (H:C-)	photodermatitis; safrole in the oil is carcinogenic; Uterine stimulant	no	PO (0.5 tsp. dried root in tea BID; many forms available)	69, 83, 278, 301, 316

See KEY and important information on p. 17-19. Abbreviations are listed on p. 163. Doses given are examples only. Read product labels carefully!

Table of Herbs and Selected Foods 93

HERB	ACTIVITY	RISKS	gras	EXAMPLE OF DOSE	REF.
echinacea	immunostimulant (A:A; H:B-C); adjuvant vs recurrent candidal vaginitis (H:B); vs URIs (H:B-); vs radiation (A:C); vs leukemia (L:C; A:C); vs colon CA (H:D); wound healing (topical) (A:B). Most studies used hydroalcohol extracts.	considered safe; Loses effectiveness after several weeks of continued use; consider intermittent use; (e.g.: 3 weeks on, 1 off)	no	PO (1 cup tea or 0.5 to 1 tsp. tincture TID—sometimes given every 2 to 3 hours for the first several doses); topical	83, 300, 301, 316
elderberry	diuretic (H:D); laxative (H:D); protects liver (A:C); vs. Influenza (H:C+); vs other viruses (H:C-D)	raw berries→nausea; leaves & stems contain some cyanide	yes*	PO ("Sambucol" is a commercially available brand; up to 1 cup tea Q 2 h on first day of illness	69, 83, 372, 406
eleuthero-coccus	adaptogenic (H:C-D); antimicrobial (L:C-D); vs CA (A:C; H:C-D) vs CAD (A:C-D); vs DM (A:B-C; H:D); protection vs radiation(L:C-D; A:C-D); ↑ T-cell immunity (H:C); prevent birth defects(A:C-D); failed to improve aerobic exercise performance (H:B; 67)	hypoglycemia (H:D)	no	PO (roots; extract) 150 mg powdered root TID	69, 83
ephedra	↓'s BP (root), ↑'s BP (above ground plant) (A:A-B; H:B); CNS stimulant (H:A); diuretic (H:A); ↑'s uterine contractions (H:B; vs asthma (H:B)	xs → dysrhythmias; xs CNS stimulation; alters DM control; possibly associated with kidney stones (538)	no	PO (adult dose: 15 mg TID)	5, 69, 83, 301, 316

See KEY and important information on p. 17-19. Abbreviations are listed on p. 163. Doses given are examples only. Read product labels carefully!

Table of Herbs and Selected Foods

HERB	ACTIVITY	RISKS	gras	EXAMPLE OF DOSE	REF.
evening primrose	source of essential fatty acids (H:A); ↓'s cholesterol (H: B); vs eczema (H:C; 147); vs diabetic neuropathy (H:C); vs fibrocystic breast dz (H:D); vs alcoholic liver dz (H:D+); vs MS (H:D); vs PMS (H:C-; 276) vs rheumatoid arthritis (H:C); to prevent headache (H:D); vs Sjogren's syndrome and systemic sclerosis (H:D; 133); vs obesity (H:D); ↓'s thrombosis(H:C)	quality of caps varies widely; "EFAMOL" is the "gold standard" Considered safe	no	PO (500 mg caps, 1 to 2 caps PO TID)	83, 133, 147, 276, 301
fennel	estrogenic (seed oil) (A:C); many traditions support GI sedative and emmenagogue effects; some traditions suggest lactagogue effect	Oil has CNS, hepatic and pulmonary toxicity; dermatitis; anticoagulant effect	yes	PO (up to 1 cup tea TID—infants would use 2 tsp. TID; caps 600 mg TID; tincture 2 ml TID)	69, 83, 301, 372, 373
fenugreek	↓'s cholesterol (A:B; H:C); ↓'s glucose (A:B; H:C); diuretic (A:C-); anti-inflammatory (A:C-D); ↓'s calcium oxalate precipitation (renal)	considered safe; (hypoglycemia H:C-D)	yes	PO (1 tsp. seeds eaten or in tea, TID)	69, 83, 301
feverfew	vs arthritis (H:C-D – see study by Pattrick which showed no benefit in rheumatoid arthritis)(227); migraine prevention (H:A); vs psoriasis (H:D)	CI-pregnancy; rebound HA on cessation; oral ulcers; ? drug interactions; not advised in infants or during lactation	no	PO 125 mg/d of dried leaves (or 2 fresh leaves/d) Leaves are eaten without cooking.	69, 83, 113, 153, 201, 227, 301
flax	↓ LDL (no Δ HDL) (H:B-); ↑ luteal phase (H:C-D); vs lupus (A:D); vs constipation (effect of fiber) (H:A)	considered safe in moderation	no	PO (seeds—2 Tbsp BID with full glass water or juice)	5, 83, 406
fo-ti	speculative uses. Cathartic (H:B)	rel. CI in pregnancy; (Is not the same as fo-ti-teng)	no	PO	69, 83, 301

See KEY and important information on p. 17-19. Abbreviations are listed on p. 163. Doses given are examples only. Read product labels carefully!

Table of Herbs and Selected Foods

HERB	ACTIVITY	RISKS	gras	EXAMPLE OF DOSE	REF.
Frankincense, Indian (Boswellia serrata)	Anti-inflammatory effects, may be useful vs. arthritis (H:C) and vs. ulcerative colitis (H:C-); to prevent anaphylaxis (A:C)	Considered safe		350 mg extract TID	83
fumitory	vs cardiac ischemia (A:C-D); vs cholecystitis or biliary colic(A:C-; H:C); vs eczema or psoriasis (H:D)	considered safe	no	PO (500 mg BID)	83; 123
galangal (alpinia)	vs anemia (A:D); antifungal (L:B); vs arthritis (A:D); vs CA (A:C); vs dementia (A:C); diuretic (A:C); vs HTN (A:C); vs male infertility (A:D)	xs → ↓ BP	yes	PO (1 g TID); topical	83
ganoderma (reishi)	vs. Chronic hepatitis B (H:C; 171); prevents altitude sickness (H:C-); vs angina (H:D+); antitumor (A:B); immunostimulant (A:B); antihistamine (A:B)	unknown	no	PO (eaten as food or taken as 1 tsp. dried powder QD to BID)	171, 369, 372, 406
garlic	↓ LDL (H:A-B); sl. ↑ HDL (H:A-B); lowers BP (H:B); antibacterial (L:B); antifungal (L:B: H:C-D); antioxidant (H:A-B); vs thrombus formation (H:A-B); vs CA (A:C-D); reviews are mixed as to comparing these effects from whole garlic vs extracts and "deodorized" garlic. Eating garlic twice/week assoc. with halving risk for prostate CA (H:C; 439).	considered safe; (long term use of extracts--?); odor (may alleviate with parsley)	yes	PO (up to 3 g powder BID; topical)	83, 301, 316, 439

See KEY and important information on p. 17-19. Abbreviations are listed on p. 163. Doses given are examples only. Read product labels carefully!

Table of Herbs and Selected Foods

HERB	ACTIVITY	RISKS	gras	EXAMPLE OF DOSE	REF.
gelsemium	analgesic and CNS depressant (H:C-)	therapeutic window too narrow; respiratory depression	no	not advised	69, 83
gentian	↑'s appetite (H:D); anti-inflammatory (A:C)	considered safe; (pregnancy ?); xs extract → n/v	yes	PO (1 g TID ac)	69, 83, 300, 301
ginger	vs nausea (H:C+); vs motion sickness (H:C+); prevents aflatoxin-related cancer (L:B)	safe		PO (500 mg powder TID)	119, 300, 301
ginkgo biloba	vs acrocyanosis (H:C+); antioxidant (H:B+); ↓'s platelet aggregation-(H:B+); vs intermittent claudication (H:C); vs PMS related breast engorgement (H:C); vs post phlebitic syndrome (H:C); vs Raynaud's (H:B-C); vs vertigo(H:C+); may help patients with Alzheimer's and vascular dementia (H:C+; 134); vs. tinnitus (H:C+; 83)	leaf extracts usu. safe; rare reports of spontaneous bleeding problems, esp. in comb. with ASA, incl. into eye or brain (249); occl vasoconstriction, GI upset or HA; severe allergies with use of whole plant may occur.	no	PO (80 to 250 mg div. BID to TID) (also IV in Europe)	57, 80, 83, 134, 249, 275, 301, 316, 332, 373-4, 406
ginseng	adaptogenic (A:B; H:C); ↑'s HDL (A:D; H:D); ↓'s glucose (H:C-); vs stress induced GI ulcer (A:B); vs post op stress (H:C-)	considered safe; occl. reports of agitation, insomnia, ↑ BP usu. involve excessive doses. AM dosing prevents insomnia.	no	PO; 1 gram of dried root per day, (3 to 8% ginsenosides)	83, 301, 316
Gluco-mannan	(= Konjac mannan); vs constipation (H:B); ↓'s LDL (H:B); ↓'s glucose (H:C+); prevention of lung CA (A:C-)	xs may → hypoglycemia; prefer caps or powder (tabs may → GI obstruction	no	PO	83

See KEY and important information on p. 17-19. Abbreviations are listed on p. 163. Doses given are examples only. Read product labels carefully!

Table of Herbs and Selected Foods

HERB	ACTIVITY	RISKS	gras	EXAMPLE OF DOSE	REF.
glucosamine	promotes cartilage repair (H:B); vs osteoarthritis (H:B+); vs post traumatic arthritis (H:C+)	probably safe (long term?); isolated report of adverse pulmonary effect (H:D)	n/a	1.5 g PO/d	83
goldenseal	antimicrobial (weak) (L:C); vs diarrhea (H:C-); vs tumors (A:C-); vs hepatic toxins (incl. etoh) (H:C-); ↓'s glucose (H:D); vs traveler's diarrhea (bourberine is active ingred.)(H:C)	CI-pregnancy; xs→ CNS toxicity; mod. doses may ↑ cardiac output and peripheral vasoconstriction	no	topical; PO with caution (500 mg TID). (bourberine 100-200 mg up to QID)	69, 83, 301, 316
gotu kola	vs bilharzia bladder lesions (IM) (H:C+); vs CA (L:D); contraceptive (A:D); vs psoriasis (topical)(H:C-); wound healing (topical application) (A:C)	considered safe; dermatitis from handling leaves	no	PO(500 mg TID); IM; topical; leaf or leaf extr. Bartram (372) advises limit therapy to 6 weeks at a time.	69, 83, 301, 316
grape seed	anti-oxidant (L:C); prevent dental caries (L:C; H:D); vs Ehrlich ascites carcinoma (A:D?); hand cleaner (oil)(H:C-); hepatoprotective (A:C)	probably safe; hepato-toxicity ? (A:D)	no	PO; topical; use of oil in cooking.	83, 316
green tea	CNS stimulant (H:A); ↓ 's incidence some tumors (H:C); ↓ LDL(H:D)	↑ glucose; ↑ cholesterol; ↑ GERD; insomnia; ↑HR } all H:A-B; ↑ incidence esoph. CA (may prevent by adding milk?)(H:C-) possibly teratogenic (A:C-; H:D); may prevent some cancers (L:B; H:C; 2)	yes	PO (1 cup tea up to TID)	2, 83
grifola	see maitake				

See KEY and important information on p. 17-19. Abbreviations are listed on p. 163. Doses given are examples only. Read product labels carefully!

Table of Herbs and Selected Foods

HERB	ACTIVITY	RISKS	gras	EXAMPLE OF DOSE	REF.
guar gum	↓'s BP (H:C); ↓'s glucose in AODM (H:B); ↓'s LDL (H:A); ↓'s wt (H:D)	considered safe; GI obstruction may occur (with tablet form primarily); xs gas (usu. improves with time)	no	PO (5 g TID but avoid tabs)	83, 372
guarana	CNS stimulant (caffeine)(H:A); ↓'s platelet aggregation (H:D+)	as for caffeine (see green tea); interaction with coumadin or aspirin?	yes	PO (up to 2 g powder per day, div. TID)	69, 83
guggul	↓'s LDL & triglycerides; ↑'s HDL } (H:B)	considered safe; GI upset.	no	PO	83
gymnema	vs DM (A:A; H:C-)	considered safe	no	PO	83, 316
hawthorn	vs angina (H:B); vs CAD (dilates coronary arteries & ↓'s PVR (H:B); vs HTN (H:A-); vs CHF(H:B; 38)	hypotension; arrhythmias	no	PO (up to 500 mg TID)	38, 69, 83, 301, 316
hibiscus	antimicrobial (L:C; A:C)	considered safe	yes	PO	83, 301
honey	vs burns (H:C); vs CA (A:D); vs cataracts (H:D); vs corneal herpes (H:D); vs PUD (active vs H.pylori)(H:C); wound healing (H:A)	allergies; CI < 1 y.o. re: botulism risk	n/a	topical; PO	83, 301
horehound	vs DM (A:C-); expectorant (H:C-)	arrhythmias with xs dose.	yes	PO	83, 301
horse chestnut	vs varicose veins (H:C+); vs arthritis (H:D)	Standardized extracts used commercially are considered safe; use of whole herb can result in fatal side effects(H:C)		topical & standardized extracts PO (caution advised)	5, 69, 83, 300, 316
horsetail	diuretic (mild) (H:B)	nicotine-like effects in xs doses.	no	PO	83, 301

See KEY and important information on p. 17-19. Abbreviations are listed on p. 163. Doses given are examples only. Read product labels carefully!

Table of Herbs and Selected Foods

HERB	ACTIVITY	RISKS	gras	EXAMPLE OF DOSE	REF.
hyssop	expectorant (H:D); vs HIV (leaf extracts)(L:C); vs pharyngitis (symptomatic relief) (H:D)	xs oil →CNS toxicity incl. seizures	yes	PO (2 g powder TID or 1 tsp. made into tea up to TID)	83, 301
jewelweed	vs poison ivy (H:D)	considered safe (topical)	no	topical	83
jojoba	vs acne (H:D); vs alopecia (H:D-); antioxidant (L:D); vs psoriasis (H:D); vs sunburn (H:D)	topical considered safe; PO- potential cardiac toxicity	no	topical (avoid PO)	83, 301
juniper	diuretic (H:B); anti-inflammatory (H:C-); vs DM (A:C); diuretic (H:C-); vs psoriasis (H:D+); wound healing (H:C-)-	allergies; potential renal dz or seizures with chronic use or in those with pre-disposing illness CI-pregnancy; allergies; diarrhea; renal toxicity; theor. Risk carcinogens from tar preparations	yes (berries)	PO (250 mg tabs TID); topical	69, 83
karaya gum	pharyngitis (symptomatic relief)(H:C-)	considered safe	yes	PO	83
kava-kava	oral anesthetic (H:B+); sedative (H:A-); anti-convulsant effects (H:C); vs. pain (H:C); vs. anxiety (H:B); mechanism may involve GABA receptor binding in the brain.	dermatitis; xs → hematuria, pulm. HTN, weakness, ↓ wbc	no	PO (2 g TID or as decoction with 30 g in 0.5 liter: 1 cup up to TID)	69, 83, 316
khat	CNS & CV stimulation (H:A-)	y dependence; CNS & CV toxicity; pulm. edema; takes place of food; altered libido	no	chewed- not adv.	69
kudzu	vs alcoholism (slows its metabolism) (A:C; H:D)	unknown	no	PO	83, 316

See KEY and important information on p. 17-19. Abbreviations are listed on p. 163. Doses given are examples only. Read product labels carefully!

Table of Herbs and Selected Foods

HERB	ACTIVITY	RISKS	gras	EXAMPLE OF DOSE	REF.
laminaria (kelp)	cervical ripening/inducing labor (H:A-)	endometritis; neonatal sepsis	no	intra-cervical	83
lavender	vs AODM (A:C; H:D); insect repellent (top.)(H:C-); vs insomnia (aroma tx)(H:D+); vs perineal pain (oil in bath)(H:C-); spasmolytic (PO)(A:C-)-	considered safe; occl. allergies or dermatitis	yes	topical; PO (one-half tsp. dried flowers made into tea—1 cup up to TID)	69, 83
lemon verbena	antibacterial (L:C)	considered safe; occl. allergies	yes	PO	83
lemongrass	essentially none	considered safe	yes	PO	83
licorice	vs arthritis (A:D); vs PUD (H:D)	may ↓ K and ↑ BP	yes	PO (2g TID)	5, 69, 83, 301, 316
linden	antibacterial (L:C; H:D); induces sweating (H:B)	cardiac toxicity with chronic use	yes	PO	69, 83, 301
lovage	diuretic (H:C-); vs. xs gas (H:C-)	considered safe; possible photodermatitis	yes	PO (1 g TID)	83, 301
mace	antibacterial (L:C); antifungal (L:C); vs CA (A:C); hepatoprotective (A:C)-	occl. allergy; overdose → dysrhythmias, hallucinations	yes	PO (750 mg TID)	83
maitake (grifola)	decreases triglycerides and total cholesterol without change in HDL (A:C; 158); to prevent or treat cancer (A:B+; H:C; 83, 204); vs diabetes (A:C; 83); vs. HTN (A:B; H:D; 83); vs obesity (A:C; H:D)	considered safe	no	PO (some studies used 500 mg of powdered maitake, once to twice per day)	83, 158, 204
marigold	see calendula				

See KEY and important information on p. 17-19. Abbreviations are listed on p. 163. Doses given are examples only. Read product labels carefully!

Table of Herbs and Selected Foods

HERB	ACTIVITY	RISKS	gras	EXAMPLE OF DOSE	REF.
marijuana	bronchodilator (short-term)(H:C); vs nausea (may be effective when other methods fail)(H:B); vs ↓ appetite in AIDS (H:C); vs MS & epilepsy (H:D+); vs glaucoma (H:D+).	intoxication; contamination (unreliable sources); may worsen seizures; ↓ PFT's with chronic use. consider Rx Marinol vs Ondansetron vs Megestrol for N/V	no	PO (R'x); smoked (where legal)	69, 83
mate'	CNS stimulant (H:B); diuretic (H:B-)	as for caffeine (CV, PUD or DM aggravation); chronic use may ↑ risk of esophageal CA	yes	PO (1 cup tea TID)	69, 83
melaleuca	antiseptic (H:C)- dental, derm, vaginal, vs UTI (PO)	occl topical irritation	yes	topical (few drops of oil topically) ; PO (not oil)	69, 83, 300, 301
melatonin	antioxidant (L:C+); vs jet lag & insomnia (H:B-); vs tumors (L:C)	considered safe; (long term ?)	n/a	PO 1 to 5 mg/d	83
milk thistle	antioxidant (H:B+); vs cirrhosis (H:C); vs viral hepatitis (H:B+); vs amanita mushroom poisoning (life saving) (H:B+; 453); vs. other hepato-toxins (H:A-)	occl allergies or GI upset; considered safe	no	PO (100 to 140 mg TID); IV (extracts)	83, 301, 316, 372, 453
mistletoe	vs tumors (extracts)(A:C); vs lung CA (H:C)	serious or fatal GI or CV effects	no	not advised (except as standardized extracts in research protocols)	83, 301, 316
monascus	Decreases LDL, VLDL and triglycerides through HMG Co-A inhibition (contains lovastatin) (H:A); may increase HDL (H:C).	Generally considered safe. Liver and muscle toxicity similar to other HMG Co-A inhibitors. Theor. SI. Risk nephrotoxicity.	83	Approx. 0.5 mg/kg per day (or as per label).	83

See KEY and important information on p. 17-19. Abbreviations are listed on p. 163. Doses given are examples only. Read product labels carefully!

Table of Herbs and Selected Foods

HERB	ACTIVITY	RISKS	gras	EXAMPLE OF DOSE	REF.
mullein	vs pharyngitis (symptomatic relief)(L:C)	considered safe	yes	PO (2 g flowers or 6 g leaves TID)	83, 301
myricetin	see bioflavonoids				
myrrh	anti-inflammatory (A:C); antimicrobial (L:C); vs DM (A:C-)	may cause uterine contractions; dermatitis	yes	PO (tincture 10 drops TID); topical	83, 301
neem	antibacterial (L:C-); contraceptive (1 ml oil per vag.)(L:B; H:D); vs DM (A:C; H:D); vs gingivitis (H:C-); insect repellent (H:A); vs PUD and gastritis (A:B; 97); vs malaria (L:C-)	LD_{50} (oil)= 15-20 ml/kg (A:C); CI in infants/small children re: potential for serious or fatal effects.	no	PO; mucosal (oil from seeds)	8; 83; 290; 193; 195; 337; 286
noni (morinda citrifolia)	mild sedative & vs. Pain (A:C; 331); vs cancer (A:C-; 128, 129)	sedation?	No	PO	128, 129, 331
nutmeg	spice only (hallucinogenic in overdose); may prevent aflatoxin-related cancer (L:B; 119); doses needed to treat diarhea or cause significant prostaglandin inhibition would put patient at risk for serious adverse effects (H:B)	in overdose (e.g., > 1 Tbsp) → intoxication, N/V/D, ↓ BP, ↓ temp	yes	PO (500 mg TID; avoid oil or use maximum of 2 drops per day)	69, 83, 119
oats	Vs. hyperlipidemia (H:B—argued whether due to specific effect or change in dietary pattern); to treat itchy rashes (H:B); adjuvant treatment of addicitons (H:C-)	Safe (may cause xs. GI gas)			83
octacosanol	ergogenic (H:D); vs Parkinson's dz (H:D)	drug interaction with levo-dopa	n/a	PO	83

See KEY and important information on p. 17-19. Abbreviations are listed on p. 163. Doses given are examples only. Read product labels carefully!

Table of Herbs and Selected Foods

HERB	ACTIVITY	RISKS	gras	EXAMPLE OF DOSE	REF.
oregano	anti-fungal (incl. Vs aflatoxin synthesis)	safe		PO	294
Pao d' Arco	see taheebo				
passion flower	antibacterial (L:C-); antifungal (L:C-); ↓ BP and dilates coronary arteries (A:C); CNS stimulant/sedative (A:C).	xs may → CNS depression	yes	PO (extracts such as 1:8 in 40% ethanol—2 ml up to QID)	83, 301, 316, 372
pectin	↓'s LDL & triglycerides (H:B+); vs radiation (GI source)(H:C)	may ↓ absorption of nutrients	n/a	PO	83
pennyroyal	none useful	severe or fatal effects may occur; stimulates abortion	yes	not advised	69, 83, 301
pepper (black)	see capsicum				
peppermint	vs irritable bowel syndrome (H:C); sm. mm. relaxant (H:C); stimulates bile (A:C)	may worsen GERD or hiatal hernia	yes	PO (1 tsp. dried leaves in 1 cup water as tea up to QID)	83, 301, 316
perilla	↓'s allergies, cholesterol, trigl., & risk of breast or colon CA}(A:C)	potential for pulmonary edema in xs dose	no	PO (leaves, seed and sprouts are edible in moderation)	69, 83
peru balsam	antimicrobial (mild)(H:C); topical/mucosal wound healing (H:C-)	occl. dermatitis; avoid on breast if breastfeeding	yes	topical; PO	83
peyote	sedative-narcotic (H:B); ↓'s blood glucose (H:C)	intoxication, hallucinations, addiction	no	PO	69

See KEY and important information on p. 17-19. Abbreviations are listed on p. 163. Doses given are examples only. Read product labels carefully!

Table of Herbs and Selected Foods

HERB	ACTIVITY	RISKS	gras	EXAMPLE OF DOSE	REF.
plantain (psyllium)	psyllium fiber: ↓'s cholesterol; vs IBS}(H:B); leaves vs poison ivy (H:D); extract- sclerosing agent (H:B)	allergies; bezoars; a potentially toxic pigment is routinely removed in processing	no	PO; topical; IV (extract)	5, 69, 83
primrose, evening	see evening primrose				
propolis	antibacterial (H:C-); anti-inflammatory (A:C); antifungal (H:C-); antioxidant (A:B); vs. CA (L:C; A:C); vs dry socket (H:C); antiviral (L:C-); vs TB (H:C-)	allergies	no	topical; PO (100 mg powder TID or standardized tinctures)	83, 301
pumpkin seeds	vs worms (GI)--(H:C); vs BPH (H:D+)	considered safe		PO (1 Tbsp seeds TID)	83, 406
pycnogenol	antioxidant (H:B); prophyl. vs connective tissue damage (A:C); vs peripheral vasc. dz (H:C)	considered safe	n/a	topical; PO	83, 316
Pygeum africanum (African plum tree)	Effective vs. benign prostatic hypertrophy	Considered safe		Extract: 50 mg BID	83
pyrethrum	insect repellent	considered safe; occl. Allergies (or wheezing with spray or vapor)		topical; spray; incense	69
quercetin	see bioflavonoids				
quillaia	vs dandruff (topical)	topical considered safe; PO- potential for severe toxicity	yes	topical; (avoid PO)	83

See KEY and important information on p. 17-19. Abbreviations are listed on p. 163. Doses given are examples only. Read product labels carefully!

Table of Herbs and Selected Foods

HERB	ACTIVITY	RISKS	gras	EXAMPLE OF DOSE	REF.
quinine	vs arrhythmias (H:A); vs leg cramps (H:B+); vs malaria (H:A); sclerosing agent (IV) (H:B)	CI- pregnancy and G6PD deficiency; ↓'s platelets (idiosyncratic); potential CNS and CV adverse effects	yes	PO	69, 83
reishi	see ganoderma				
rose hips	vitamin C source (H:A-); laxative (H:B)	considered safe	yes	PO (1 tsp. in 1 cup water as tea)	83, 301
rosemary	antioxidant (L:C); prevents breast CA (A:C); insect repellent (L:C)	allergies; xs use of oil → GI and renal toxicity	yes	PO (as spice or 1 tsp. in 1 cup water as tea); topical	69, 83, 301
royal jelly	antimicrobial (L:D+); vs CA (A:D)	allergies	n/a	PO; topical	83, 301
rue	antimicrobial (L:C); causes abortion (H:C); ↓'s GI & coronary spasms); potential CNS and CV adverse effects; artery spasms (A:C)	CI- pregnancy; oil- mutagenic (L:C); xs → sev. hepato-renal toxicity	yes	PO (500 mg TID); topical (risks>benefits)	69, 301
safflower	vs fever (tea)(H:D+); laxative (oil)(H:C); ↓'s LDL (oil)(H:C); good source of essential fatty acids (H:A)	considered safe	no	PO	83
saffron	vs CA (L:C; A:D+); ↓'s cholesterol & trigl. (A:C); ↑'s O2 diffusion in plasma (L:B) which → lower risk CV dz (H:D+)	considered safe in usu. amt.; large xs → CNS sedation or even death	yes	PO (10 drops tincture TID); oil from stigmus of flower)	69, 83
sage	antimicrobial (L:C); antioxidant (L:B-); antispasmotic (GI)(A:C)	considered safe. Bartram (372) advises to avoid in HTN, epilepsy and pregnancy.	yes	PO (500 mg TID)	69, 83, 301

See KEY and important information on p. 17-19. Abbreviations are listed on p. 163. Doses given are examples only. Read product labels carefully!

Table of Herbs and Selected Foods

HERB	ACTIVITY	RISKS	gras	EXAMPLE OF DOSE	REF.
sandalwood	diuretic (H:D); vs UTI (H:D-)	dermatitis	yes	PO (3 drops oil TID)	69, 83
sassafras	antimicrobial (L:C); induces sweating (H:C); vs insect bites and stings (topical)(H:D)	carcinogenic (A:B); xs oil (e.g. 5 ml)→ CNS toxicity	yes	not advised	69, 83, 301
savory	anti-diuretic (H:D); antimicrobial (L:C); aphrodisiac (summer)(H:D-); GI spasmolytic (H:D+); ↓'s libido (winter)(H:D-)	considered safe	yes	PO	83, 301
saw palmetto	vs allergies (A:C-); anti-inflammatory (A:D+); vs BPH (H:B)	CI-pregnancy; xs → diarrhea; occl HA; theor. risk of aggravation of estrogen-sensitive tumors	no	PO (300 mg extract or 2 g seeds per day, div. BID)	34, 69, 300, 301, 316, 406
schisandra	anti-tussive (A:C); hepatoprotective (L:D); vs TB (L:D+)	CNS depression; potential drug interactions and mutagenicity	no	PO-not advised	83, 301
scullcap	antibacterial and antifungal (L:C-); vs CA (A:D); vs HTN (A:D)	xs→ mental status changes and seizure-like activity	no	PO (1 tsp. in 1 cup water as tea up to TID)	83, 301, 373
senna	laxative (H:A)	dependency with chronic use; melanosis coli; clubbed nails	yes	PO	5, 69, 83, 301
shark cartilage	antibacterial, anti-protozoa and anti-fungal (extracts)(L:C); vs CA (H:D-)	unknown	n/a	PO	83
shiitake mushroom	antiviral (prophylactic-intranasal)(A:C-); ↓'s cholesterol (PO)(A: C-); vs colon CA (T-cell mech.)(H:C-)	considered safe	no	PO (food); IV (extract: lentinan)	47, 83, 316

See KEY and important information on p. 17-19. Abbreviations are listed on p. 163. Doses given are examples only. Read product labels carefully!

Table of Herbs and Selected Foods 107

HERB	ACTIVITY	RISKS	gras	EXAMPLE OF DOSE	REF.
silymarin	see bioflavonoids and milk thistle				
slippery elm	vs herpes (H:D); vs pharyngitis (symptomatic)(H:D+)	allergies	no	PO (lozenges) wide safety margin	69, 83
soapwort	vs poison ivy (H:D)	N/V/D with PO use	no	topical only	83
soy	Protein source (H:A); vs menopausal symptoms (H:B); preventative vs. breast and prostate cancer (H:B); vs. BPH (L:B).	Inhalation of dust may cause bronchospasm		45 g per day of soy (or isoflavone extracts—per label or about 100 mg per day)	83
spirulina	protein, vitamin and mineral source (H:B); regression of oral leukoplakia in tobacco chewers (H:C); vs. other neoplasms (A:C)	occl heavy metal contamination; cost inefficient; content of true vit. B-12 doubtful	no	PO	83, 301
squill	vs CA (L:C); vs dandruff (topical)(H:D); expectorant (H:C+); peripheral vasodilatation & bradycardia (A:B; H:C-)	narrow therapeutic window; (CV & GI toxicity); red squill-CNS toxicity.	no	PO- not advised	5, 83
St. John's Wort	antidepressant (H:B) mechanism: inhibits serotonin re-uptake (A:B) & may affect GABA receptors (513). Role of MAO inhibiton likely minimal (L:C); antiviral (A:C); vs HIV (H:D); vs vitiligo (H:C-); antibacterial (L:C)	photodermatitis; high in tannins. (theor. CA risk); consider possible interactions as with MAO-I drugs as well as those affecting serotonin	yes	PO: whole herb: 3 g TID or 1 tsp. in 1 cup water as tea, BID to TID; standard extract (0.3% hypericin): 300 mg TID	69, 82, 83, 300, 301, 316, 373, 406, 513
Stinging nettle	Leaf extracts-- anti-inflammatory effect during bladder irrigation (H:C); root extract—taken orally effective vs. BPH (H:C); vs. HIV and CMV (L:C).	Allergies (and topical stinging from skin contact with mature plants); may elevate blood glucose		Per labels (herbal preps typically 5 to 10 grams/day in divided doses)	5, 83

See KEY and important information on p. 17-19. Abbreviations are listed on p. 163. Doses given are examples only. Read product labels carefully!

Table of Herbs and Selected Foods

HERB	ACTIVITY	RISKS	gras	EXAMPLE OF DOSE	REF.
storax (styrax)	antibacterial (topical)(H:D); vs pharyngitis (symptomatic)(H:D)	allergies; theor. risk re: tannins	yes	topical; PO	83
taheebo	antimicrobial (L:C); vs CA (H:D-)	xs → severe or fatal toxicity	no	top.; PO-not adv.	83
tansy	antibacterial (L:C-); antispasmotic (H:D); vs tick-borne encephalitis virus (A:C-)-	reports of severe and fatal reactions	yes	not advised	69, 301
tea tree	see melaleuca				
Terminalia arjuna	Versus CHF (H:B)	Uncertain; no apparent adverse effects in early studies.		500 mg extract every 8 hours (PO)	515
tofu—see soy					
tolu balsam	antiseptic (mild-topical)(H:C-); expectorant (mild)(H:C-)	occl allergies	yes	PO; topical	83
tomato	↓ risk prostate CA (H:B-; 429, 430)	occl allergies		PO	69, 429, and 430
tonka bean	vs schistosomiasis (H:D-)	potential for severe hepatotoxicity in large doses	no	not advised	69, 83
tragacanth	vs CA (L:C-; A:D+); vs DM (H:D); vs cough/cold symptoms (H:D)	considered safe	yes	PO (1 g powder TID)	83, 372
trillium	antifungal (L:C); vs bleeding (topical-H:C-; PO- H:D-); vs diarrhea (H:C-)	topical considered safe; PO- probably safe in small amts.; xs → potential cardiac toxicity	no	top.; PO-not adv.	83

See KEY and important information on p. 17-19. Abbreviations are listed on p. 163. Doses given are examples only. Read product labels carefully!

Table of Herbs and Selected Foods

HERB	ACTIVITY	RISKS	gras	EXAMPLE OF DOSE	REF.
turmeric	antioxidant (A:A; H:B); vs arthritis (A:C-); prevention of CA (A:B; H:C); tx of CA (H:D-); hepatoprotective (A:A; H:C); vs scabies (topical)(H:C+); platelet inhibition (L:B; 288)	considered safe	yes	PO (250 to 500 mg BID); topical	83, 316, 406
turpentine (pine oil)	antibacterial (L:C-); counterirritant (H:D); wound debridement (H: D)	potential severe or fatal toxicity	yes	not advised	83
unicorn root	see aletris				
uva ursi	mild diuretic (H:B); vs UTI (requires alkaline urine)(L:C)	CI- pregnancy; tannins; considered safe in small amts. but potential for severe or fatal toxicity in xs.	no	PO (1 tsp. in 1 cup water as tea TID)	5, 83, 301
valerian	vs HTN (A:D); vs insomnia (H:B); sedative (H:B); vs seizures (A: D)	considered safe; long-term? pregnancy?	yes	PO (take 1 hr before bedtime for insomnia) (1 tsp. dried root as tea or 160 to 800 mg powder as caps per dose)	69, 83, 100, 301, 316, 372
vanilla	aphrodisiac (H:D+); caries prevention (H:D); ↑'s satiety	occl allergies	yes	PO; aroma	69, 83
vitex	see chaste tree				
white cohosh	none useful	CNS, CV & GI toxicity	no	not advised	83

See KEY and important information on p. 17-19. Abbreviations are listed on p. 163. Doses given are examples only. Read product labels carefully!

Table of Herbs and Selected Foods

HERB	ACTIVITY	RISKS	gras	EXAMPLE OF DOSE	REF.
wine (red)	↑ HDL (H:A-B); antioxidant (H:B-C); inhibits platelet aggregation (H:B-C); ↑gastric emptying (H:C-D) (white wine); may decrease risk of Alzheimer's disease (H:C; 600, 601); vs polio (L:C-)	avoid MAO-I; 10% risk alcoholism; may worsen GERD; tannins		PO 4-8 oz/d	83
wintergreen	digestive aid (H:D); topical analgesic (H:C)	xs PO is toxic (esp. in children)	no	topical; PO-?	69, 83
witch hazel	vs bleeding (topical)(H:C-); vs varicose vv (H:D-)	uncertain; theor. risk re: carcinogens (high in tannins)	no	top.; PO-not adv.	69, 83, 301
withania	anti-inflammatory (A:C); hepato-protective (A:D); sedative (A:D); vs stress (A:C-); anti-tumor and radiosensitizing effects (L:B; A:B)	possible CNS depression; LD_{50} = 1g/kg (A:C)	no	PO	63, 83
woodruff	antibacterial (H:D); anti-inflammatory (A:D+); wound healing (topical)(H:D-)	considered safe	yes	top.; PO (1 tsp. in 1 cup water as tea BID)	69, 83
wormwood	antihelminth (H:C)	neuro-toxic	y/n	not advised	83, 301
Yams (wild)	Alleviates PMS and menopausal symptoms (H:D, 278)			PO (and commercial cream preparations)	278
yarrow	anti-inflammatory (A:C); antimicrobial (L:C); vs bleeding (topical) (H:C-); wound healing (H:C-); vs CA (A:C)	occl allergies; considered safe	yes	topical; PO (1 tsp. in 1 cup water as tea TID)	69, 83
yeast	see "brewer's yeast"				

See KEY and important information on p. 17-19. Abbreviations are listed on p. 163. Doses given are examples only. Read product labels carefully!

Table of Herbs and Selected Foods

HERB	ACTIVITY	RISKS	gras	EXAMPLE OF DOSE	REF.
yellow dock	laxative (H:D); vs CA (L:D)	high in tannins; high in oxalates (kidney stone risk)—↓'ed with boiling and rinsing before use.	no	PO (boil & rinse first—3 g TID)	69, 83, 301
yellow root	antibacterial (L:D); vs DM (H:0); vs HTN (H:D+)	considered safe; (one case of arsenic contamination)	no	PO	83
yerba santa	vs bruises (H:0); expectorant (H:D)	considered safe	yes	topical; PO	83
yew	extract (paclitaxel, et al) effective vs CA (H:A-)	bone marrow suppression; cardiac toxicity	no	IV (R'x)	83, 300
yohimbe	vs erectile dysfunction (H:C+); aphrodisiac (H:D).	anxiety; CNS stimulation; direct effect is to lower BP, however, since it is a MAO-I it can increase BP via interaction with other herbs, drugs or food.	no	PO (5 mg TID)	69, 83, 301, 598
yucca	vs arthritis (H:D); vs CMV (L:C-); vs herpes (L:C-); vs HTN (H:D); vs melanoma (A:D+); migraine prevention (H:D)	considered safe	yes	PO	83, 301, 316

See KEY and important information on p. 17-19. Abbreviations are listed on p. 163. Doses given are examples only. Read product labels carefully!

TABLE OF NUTRIENTS

Name of nutrient	Essential?	Benefits	Risks	Sources	RDA
Arsenic	Possibly (mineral)	methionine metabolism	a potent, life-threatening poison in anything but trace amounts	unknown (trace)	unknown (12 to 25 mcg?)(305)
Biotin	yes (vitamin)	metabolism of CHO, fat and protein. Deficiency is rare. Raw egg white binds biotin. Dermatitis and muscle weakness or pain reported in deficiency states.	Essentially none.	Egg yolk, yeast, dairy, legumes.	30 to 100 mcg
Boron	probably	bone growth (synergistic with Vitamin D) (A:B; 135; 210)	unknown; (OSHA standards exist for excess occupational exposure—see Moore J)	water, variety of foods (varies with soil content)	unknown (trace amounts) Avoid over 7.5 mg/d? (196)

See KEY and important information on p. 17-19; abbreviations- p. 163

Nutrient	Essential?	Activity	Risks	Sources	RDA
Bromine	possibly	unknown (see 305)	unknown	unknown	unknown
Cadmium	possibly	unknown (see 305; 210)	toxic in xs.	environmental	unknown
Calcium	yes	muscle contraction, nerve conduction, bone and teeth formation, blood clotting ("factor 4"). Effective vs. PMS (H:B; 470) and, along with linoleic acid, may prevent preeclampsia (H:B; 539). The following are associated with increased calcium need: high protein diets, high intake of soda drinks, and regular use of H-2 blockers.	Excess may interfere with absorption of other minerals; kidney stones in susceptible individuals	milk, cheese, yogurt, calcium set tofu, dark green vegetables (not spinach re: phytates); almonds, shrimp, molasses, bones.	800 to 1500 mg (1200 mg elemental calcium ever day, as calcium carbonate, was used in the PMS study)

See KEY and important information on p. 17-19; abbreviations- p. 163

Nutrient	Essential?	Activity	Risks	Sources	RDA
Chloride	yes (mineral)	acid-base balance	rare or unknown	as for sodium	presumed adequate when sodium intake OK
Chromium	yes (mineral)	glucose metabolism. May prevent or improve some cases of diabetes (esp. elderly with deficient or highly refined diets) (H:C+; 186, 468). Unless deficient in this, not likely to help otherwise healthy people lose excess fat or gain lean muscle. (H:C;186)	Use in diabetics requires supervision (risk for hypoglycemia—medication may need adjusting); long term excess may lead to DNA damage (A:C; H:C-; 283)	wheat germ, whole grains, brewer's yeast, meats.	50 to 200 mcg

See KEY and important information on p. 17-19; abbreviations- p. 163

Nutrient	Essential?	Activity	Risks	Sources	RDA
Copper	yes (mineral)	collagen and rbc formation; bone strength; aids iron absorption.	Neurologic and GI symptoms with excess intake or error in metabolism (Wilson's disease)	shellfish, nuts, legumes	1.5 to 3 mg
Essential fatty acids	yes	see linoleic and linolenic acid			
Fluoride	yes (mineral)	prevents tooth decay; may help prevent osteoporosis	excess leads to discoloration of teeth; popular fear of disease from appropriate fluoridation is unsupported by our review of data (H:A; 466, 467)	water (naturally in some areas; added in some areas); fish, tea.	1.5 to 4 mg

Nutrient	Essential?	Activity	Risks	Sources	RDA
Folic acid (folate; folacin)	yes (vitamin)	needed to make new cells, including blood cells; (DNA & RNA synthesis); needed for normal development of fetus (deficiency strongly associated with spina bifida or neural tube defects); decreases risk for CAD by decreasing homocysteine levels	excess may interfere with other nutrients or prescription drugs; excess also masks B12 deficiency	green leafy vegetables, oranges, legumes, seeds, beets, broccoli, wheat germ, brewer's yeast; fortified cereals and grain products.	200 to 400 mcg
German- ium	possibly (mineral)	may aid in bone formation	unknown but probably not good	unknown (trace)	unknown (trace)
Iodine	yes (mineral)	thyroid hormone production	excess may cause an acne-like rash	iodized salt; seafood; vegetables grown in coastal areas	150 mcg

See KEY and important information on p. 17-19; abbreviations- p. 163

Nutrient	Essential?	Activity	Risks	Sources	RDA
Iron	yes (mineral)	hemoglobin synthesis; needed by several enzymes in variety of metabolic pathways; can effectively treat restless legs syndrome (when iron deficiency is present).	supplements often cause upset stomach and constipation. Excess (even from foods alone) can cause hemochromatosis with its fatigue, GI and heart problems. Iron pills accidentally taken in overdose by children is a common life-threatening medical emergency.	Meats, legumes, nuts, green leafy vegetables, oysters, clams, molasses; fortified cereals and grain products.	10 to 15 mg
Lead	possibly	unknown (see 305; 210)	CNS toxicity; growth delay	environmental	unknown

See KEY and important information on p. 17-19; abbreviations- p. 163

Nutrient	Essential?	Activity	Risks	Sources	RDA
Linoleic acid	yes	multiple, esp. membrane synthesis; used to make arachidonic acid, which is found in membrane phospholipid layers. Linoleic acid is an omega-6 fatty acid. (H:A; 138); may prevent preeclampsia (H:B; 539)	unknown	vegetable oils—esp. seed oils such as grape seed oil. (safflower oil is high in linoleic acid). Meats contain arachidonic acid.	?

See KEY and important information on p. 17-19; abbreviations- p. 163

Nutrient	Essential?	Activity	Risks	Sources	RDA
Linolenic acid	yes	multiple, including eye and brain health; has role in cancer prevention (A:B+; 469). From linolenic acid (an omega-3 fatty acid), the body slowly makes eicosapentaenoic acid (EPA) and docosahexaenoic acid (DHA). (H:A; 138)	unknown	leafy green vegetables and vegetable oils. (Fish is best direct source of EPA and DHA); flax seed oil.	?
Lithium	possibly (mineral)	has been used successfully in trials vs. Cluster headaches (H:C+; 317)	excess can cause heart dysrhythmias as well as lesser problems (assoc. with carpal tunnel syndrome and with seborheic type of dermatitis—317)	unknown (trace)	unknown (trace amounts)

See KEY and important information on p. 17-19; abbreviations- p. 163

Nutrient	Essential?	Activity	Risks	Sources	RDA
Magnesium	yes (mineral)	multiple, including bone and teeth formation, energy metabolism, muscle relaxation, regulation of blood calcium levels. Used to treat some heart rhythm disorders, (esp. in deficiency states), and some complications of pregnancy (esp. pre-term labor and pre-eclampsia). Often added (with Vit. B1) to initial treatment for alcoholics. May alleviate headaches.	Excess leads to muscle weakness and ultimately paralysis, (including of respiratory muscles).	Green leafy vegetables, legumes, whole grains, molasses, nuts, seeds, and chocolate!	280 to 400 mg

See KEY and important information on p. 17-19; abbreviations- p. 163

Nutrient	Essential?	Activity	Risks	Sources	RDA
Manga-nese	yes (mineral)	Various metabolic functions, including bone and connective tissue formation.	Neuro-toxic in chronic excess. Excess also has been associated with increased risk of prostate cancer (H:C-; 203)	nuts, legumes, tea, coffee	2 to 5 mg
Molybde-num	yes (mineral)	needed for various metabolic pathways	excess leads to joint pains	legumes, liver, green leafy vegetables, wheat germ. (Does vary with soil content)	75 to 250 mcg
Nickel	probably	DNA function or transport? (210, 305)	GI and neuro toxicity	unknown (trace)	unknown (100 mcg?)(305)

See KEY and important information on p. 17-19; abbreviations- p. 163

Nutrient	Essential?	Activity	Risks	Sources	RDA
Phosphorous	yes (mineral)	energy metabolism (e.g., ATP); DNA, bone and teeth formation	excess interferes with calcium use, (e.g.. In growing teenagers who drink too many sodas)	dairy, meats, legumes, nuts, cola beverages	800 to 1200 mg
Potassium	yes (mineral)	muscle and nerve function, (including regulation of heart rhythm)	excess can cause fatal heart dysrhythmias, (usually relevant only when kidney function is impaired and/or medications are affecting its use or elimination)	potatoes, bananas, citrus fruits, dried fruits, cantaloupe, milk, yogurt, molasses, clams, crab, oysters, meats.	2 to 3 g
Rubidium	possibly	unknown (see 305)	unknown	unknown	unknown

See KEY and important information on p. 17-19; abbreviations- p. 163

Nutrient	Essential?	Activity	Risks	Sources	RDA
Selenium	yes (mineral)	antioxidant; optimum amounts (neither too little nor too much) may prevent some cancers.	GI and neuro toxicity, including death	Brazil nuts (3 nuts about = total daily need for Se); fish, some vegetables (depends upon content in soil)	55 to 70 mcg
Silicon	possibly	stimulates bone growth (A:B;263)	Unknown (pulmonary silicosis well documented in cases of chronic excess inhalation of silicates)	ubiquitous?	unknown (2 to 5 mg?) (305)

See KEY and important information on p. 17-19; abbreviations- p. 163

Nutrient	Essential?	Activity	Risks	Sources	RDA
Sodium	yes (mineral)	nerve conduction; kidney function and blood pressure regulation; deficiency unusual but may occur with heavy sweating, replaced with water—muscle cramps and headache may occur.	Excess raises blood pressure in some persons (about a third of individuals)	baked grains, table salt; pickled vegetables, cheese, canned foods, soy sauce, meats.	We need about 500 m; but avg. intake in US/ is 4 g
Sulfur	yes (mineral)	multiple, including skin, hair and nail formation and many metabolic processes	unknown from foods	most protein sources	presumed adequate when protein intake OK
Tin	possibly (mineral)	unknown (co-enzyme?)	unknown but probably not good	unknown (trace)	unknown (trace amounts)

See KEY and important information on p. 17-19; abbreviations- p. 163

Nutrient	Essential?	Activity	Risks	Sources	RDA
Vana-dium	possibly (mineral)	cofactor for some enzymes; (A:A; H:B-; 118, 210)	Unknown but probably not good	ubiquitous (trace amounts)	unknown (avg. US: 30 to 50 mcg) (118)
Vitamin A	yes (vitamin)	eyes, skin, multiple	fat soluble. Multiple, incl. HA, fatigue, birth defects	yellow, orange or dark green vegetables; apricots, cantaloupe, milk (fortified), liver, fish oil	F: 800 mcg RE; M: 1000 mcg RE
Vitamin B1 (thia-mine)	yes (vitamin)	CHO utilization; nerve function; (dramatic improvement in some alcoholics—esp. re: Wernicke's encephalopathy); beri beri (incl. CHF)	rare? (water soluble)	pork, whole grains and cereals (esp. if fortified); peas; brewer's yeast, sunflower seeds	1.0 to 1.5 mg

See KEY and important information on p. 17-19; abbreviations- p. 163

Nutrient	Essential?	Activity	Risks	Sources	RDA
Vitamin B2 (riboflavin)	yes (vitamin)	to obtain energy from food. Eye function and health of mucous membranes.	Excess may interfere with other B vitamins	Nuts and seeds, meats, dairy, mushrooms, oysters, pork.	1.2 to 1.8 mg
Vitamin B3 (niacin)	yes (vitamin)	to obtain energy from food; GI, skin and nerve function. (Pellagra is deficiency state which manifests as dermatitis of sun exposed skin, diarrhea, dementia). In high doses lowers LDL and raises HDL (with side effects potential).	Hot flushes and itching common; liver damage	meats, fish, nuts, peanuts, mushrooms, fortified cereals and grains.	13 to 20 mg

See KEY and important information on p. 17-19; abbreviations- p. 163

Nutrient	Essential?	Activity	Risks	Sources	RDA
Vitamin B5 (pantothenic acid)	yes (vitamin)	to obtain energy from foods. (Part of coenzyme A), deficiency never documented except under experimental conditions	excess may cause diarrhea	most foods (except canned)	4 to 7 mg

See KEY and important information on p. 17-19; abbreviations- p. 163

Nutrient	Essential?	Activity	Risks	Sources	RDA
Vitamin B6 (pyridoxine)	yes (vitamin)	metabolism of amino acids; immune (antibody formation), rbc and nerve functions; may have role in atherosclerosis prevention. May help some with carpal tunnel like symptoms, PMS or hyperemesis gravidarum (H:C-D; 68, 75, 287)	Large excess (on order of 500 mg daily) may cause nerve damage. (H:B; Parry G)	bananas, wheat germ, meat, fish, potatoes, brewer's yeast, fortified breakfast cereals.	1.6 to 2.2 mg

See KEY and important information on p. 17-19; abbreviations- p. 163

Nutrient	Essential?	Activity	Risks	Sources	RDA
Vitamin B12 (cyanocobalamin)	yes (vitamin)	rbc formation and nerve function. Those with GI malabsorption (or removal of large parts of stomach or distal small bowel) or strict vegetarians may be vulnerable.	Essentially none.	All animal products, including dairy and fish; some fortified foods.	2 to 2.6 mcg

See KEY and important information on p. 17-19; abbreviations- p. 163

Nutrients

Nutrient	Essential?	Activity	Risks	Sources	RDA
Vitamin C (ascorbic acid)	yes (vitamin)	Needed for integrity of collagen. Is an antioxidant. Aids in absorption of iron. Deficiency leads to delayed wound healing, bleeding gums, and poor bone formation. (Scurvy).	Diarrhea, possibly kidney stones, worsening of gout; may precipitate sickle cell crisis. When 500 mg per day or more is taken, vitamin C actually oxidizes adenine to oxoadenine, a potentially deleterious change in this DNA building block. (537)	Citrus fruits, cantaloupe, guava, kiwi, strawberry, broccoli, fresh red or green peppers, mango, papaya, Brussels sprouts.	60 to 95 mg Optimum 100-200mg/d (more under stress) (H:C; 105)

See KEY and important information on p. 17-19; abbreviations- p. 163

Nutrient	Essential?	Activity	Risks	Sources	RDA
Vitamin D	yes (vitamin, but we can make it ourselves with sun exposure)	bone and teeth development. Deficiency leads to weak bones, (classically "rickets").	Excess leads to diarrhea, headache, and abnormal deposition of calcium in tissues.	Sun exposure (at latitudes under 40 degrees), fortified milk, fish oil, liver, many calcium supplements, fortified cereal, egg yolk.	5 to 10 mcg
Vitamin E (tocopherol)	yes (vitamin)	antioxidant; rbc formation; may help prevent coronary heart disease; often successful vs. Nocturnal leg cramps (H:B+; 317)	Excess may lead to bleeding problems. Can increase effect of coumadin.	Wheat germ, seeds, nuts, plant oils, dark green leafy vegetables	8 to 12 mg (12 to 18 IU)

See KEY and important information on p. 17-19; abbreviations- p. 163

Nutrient	Essential?	Activity	Risks	Sources	RDA
Vitamin K	yes? (Also made by bacteria in our intestines)	needed for blood clotting, it is relatively deficient the first few days of life. Needed for calcium regulation.	Excess may lead to bleeding. Jaundice (water soluble forms). Counteracts effects of coumadin.	green leafy vegetables, broccoli, liver.	45 to 80 mcg
Zinc	yes (mineral)	Deficiency is associated with stunted growth, poor wound healing, altered and impaired taste, increased risk of prostatitis and prostate cancer, and both male and female infertility (H:A to C-; 71; 18).	Over 50 mg per day is associated with lowering of HDL, (also reported as when Zn:Cu intake is over 17:1). (H:B; Black, et al). Excess is associated with increased risk of benign prostate enlargement (H:C; 71)	oysters, clams, meats, whole grains (when leavened with yeast), fish	12 to 15 mg

FAVORITE WEB SITES

Data bases:

1. Centers for Disease Control: **http://www.cdc.gov**
2. Doctor's guide to the internet: **http://www.pslgroup.com/docguide.htm**
3. FDA: **http://www.fda.gov/fdahomepage.html**
4. National Library of Medicine: **http://www.ncbi.nlm.nih.gov/PubMed**
5. Physicians' choice medical web site reviews: **http://www.mdchoice.com**
6. Tufts university nutrition navigator: **http://www.navigator.tufts.edu**

Complementary therapy organizations (and their critics):
1. **American Massage Therapy Association:** http://www.AMTAMASSAGE.org
2. **Boitumelo Publishing, Inc.** (Provides a bulletin board posting reviews of current issues in alternative and complementary medicine): http://www.boitumelo.com
3. Focus on alternative and complementary therapies (FACT)— **Exeter University's Dept. of Complementary Medicine: http://www.ex.ac.uk/FACT/**
4. Herb Research Foundation: **http://www.herbs.org**
5. Homeopathic Education Service: **http://www.homeopathic.com**
6. National Certif. Bureau for Therapeutic Massage and Bodywork: **http://www.ncbtmb.com**
7. National Council For Reliable Health Information: **http://www.ncahf.org** and **http://www.quackwatch.org**
8. Univ. of Arizona, Program in Integrative Medicine: **http://www.ahsc.arizona.edu/integrative_medicine**

Patient education (screened for reliability):

1. Agency for Health Care Policy and Research/Consumer Health: **http://www.ahcpr.gov:80/consumer**

2. American Cancer Society: **http://www.cancer.org**
3. Doc in the Box: **http://www.onlinedoc.com**
4. Johns Hopkins Medical Institutions InfoNet/Patient advocacy page: **http://infonet.welch.jhu.edu/advocacy.html**

5. Medical Matrix/Patient Education: **http://www.slackinc.com/matrix/index.html**

6. MedicineNet: **http://www.medicinenet.com**
7. RxList:interaction check of most common meds: **http://www.rxlist.com/interact.html**

8. Travel Information— (**CDC**): **http://www.cdc.gov**
9. US National Library of Medicine: **http://www.nlm.gov**

References

1. Adams M, Houpt K, Cruz PD Jr. Is **phototherapy** safe for HIV-infected individuals? Photochem Photobiol 1996; 64(2):234-7
2. Agarwal R, Mukhtar H. Cancer chemoprevention by polyphenols in **green tea** and **artichoke**. Adv Exp Med Biol 1996; (401):35-50.
3. Aldridge D. Alzheimer's disease: rhythm, timing and **music** as therapy. Biomed Pharmacother 1994; 48(7):275-81.
4. Alpha-tocopherol, beta carotene cancer prevention study group. The effect of **vitamin E and beta carotene** on the incidence of lung cancer . . . NEJM 1994;330:1029-35.
5. American Botanical Council. German **Commission E Monographs**, (engl. tr). Austin, TX: American Botanical Council, 1998.
6. Amorde-Spalding K, Woch M. Rediscovering the benefits of **ketogenic diet** therapy for children. J AM Diet. Assoc. 1996;96(11):1134-5.
7. Andrade L, Ferraz M, et al. A randomized controlled trial to evaluate the effectiveness of **homeopathy** in rheumatoid arthritis. Scan J Rheum 1991;20(3):204-8
8. Ansari M, Razdan R. Operational feasibility of malaria control by burning **neem oil** in kerosene lamp in Beel Akbarpur village, District Ghaziabad, India. Indian J Malariol 1996; 33(2):81-7.
9. Baillargeon L, Drouin J, et al. The effects of **arnica montana** on blood coagulation. Can Fam Physician 1993; 39:2362-7.
10. Baker M. The **force** may be with you. Stanford Medicine 1996; 13(4):18-22.
11. Balachandran B, Sivaramkrishnan V. Induction of tumours by **Indian dietary** constituents. Indian J Cancer 1995; 32(3):104-9.
12. Bao Z. Amelioration of aminoglycoside nephrotoxicity by **Cordyceps sinensis** in old patients. Chung Kuo Chung His I Chieh Ho Tsa Chih 1994; 14(5):271-3.
13. Baram D. **Hypnosis** in reproductive health care a review and case reports. Birth 1995; 22(1):37-42
14. Barefoot J, Schroll M. Symptoms of **depression, acute myocardial infarction**, and total mortality in a community sample. Circulation. 1996; 93(11):1976-80.
15. Barrett S, Jarvis W, Kroger M, London W. *Consumer Health: A Guide to Intelligent Decisions.* Madison, WI: Brown & Benchmark, Publishers, 1997. (Sixth editon).
16. Bauer M, Gauer G, et al. Evaluation of **immune parameters in depressed** patients. Life Sci 1995; 57(7):665-74
17. Bauer R, Wagner H. **Echinacea** species as potential immunostimulatory drugs. Econ Med Plant Res. 1991; 5:253-321.
18. Bedwal R, Bahuguna A. **Zinc, copper and selenium** in reproduction. Experientia. 1994; 50(7):626-40
19. Belin P, Van Eeckhout P, et al. Recovery from nonfluent aphasia after **melodic intonation** therapy: a PET study. Neurology 1996; 47(6):1504-11.
20. Bell I, Edman J, et al. **B complex vitamin** patterns in geriatric and young adult inpatients with major depression. J Am Geriatr Soc 1991; 39(3):252-7.

21. Benoni G, Bellavite P, et al. Changes in several neutrophil functions in **basketball** players . . . Int J Sports Med 1995; 16(1):34-7
22. Berrio L; Polansky M; Anderson R. Insulin activity: stimulatory effects of **cinnamon and brewer's yeast** as influenced by albumin. Horm Res 1992; 37(6):225-9.
23. Bhatia S, Kochar N, et al. **Lactobacillus acidophilus** inhibits growth of Campylobacter pylori in vitro. J Clin Microbiol 1989; 27(10):2328-30.
24. Black M, Medeiros D, et al. **Zinc** supplements and serum lipids in young adult white males. Am J Clin Nutr 1988; 47:970-5.
25. Blot W, Li J, et al. **Nutrition intervention** trials in Linxian, China: . . . J Natl Cancer Inst. 1993; 85:1483-92.
26. Blumenstein B, Bar-eli M, et al. The augmenting role of **biofeedback** . . . J Sports Sci 1995; 13(4):343-54.
27. Boffa M, Gilmour E, Ead R. **Celery** soup causing severe phototoxicity during PUVA therapy. Br J Dermatol 1996; 135(2):334.
28. Boik J. **Cancer and Natural Medicine.** Princeton, MN: Oregon Medical Press, 1995.
29. Bokemeyer C. **Silibinin** protects against cisplatin-induced nephrotoxicity without compromising cisplatin or ifosfamide anti-tumor activity. Br J Cancer 1996; 74(12):2036-41.
30. Bol'shakova IV, Lozovskaia E, Sapezhinskii II. Antioxidant properties of a series of extracts from **medicinal plants**. Biofizika 1997; 42(2):480-3.
31. Boris M, Mandel F. Foods and additives are common causes of the **attention deficit hyperactive disorder** in children. Ann Allergy 1994; 72(5):462-8.
32. Boulos Z, Campbell S, et al. **Light treatment** for sleep disorders: . . . J Biol Rhythms 1995; 10(2):167-76
33. Boxer M, Roberts M, Grammer L. **Cumin** anaphylaxis: a case report. J Allergy Clin Immunol 1997; 99(5):722-3.
34. Bracher F. Phytotherapy of benign **prostatic hyperplasia**. Urologe A 1997; 36(1):10-7.
35. Braunig B, et al. **Echinacea** purpurea radix for strengthening the immune response in flu-like infections. Zeitschr Phytother. 1992; 13:7-13.
36. Brewer C. Second-line and 'alternative' treatments for **alcohol withdrawl** . . . Alsohol Alcohol 1995; 30(6):799-803
37. Brezinka V, Kittel F. **Psychosocial factors of coronary heart disease** in women: a review. Soc Sci Med 1996; 42(10):1351-65.
38. Brown, DJ. European Phytomedicines: research updates on chemistry, pharmacology, and clinical applications. Herbal Gram 1997; 39:62-66.
39. Bruhn C, Wood OB. Position of the American Dietetic Association: **food irradiation**. J Am Diet Assoc. 1996; 96(1):69-72.
40. Burke M, Walsh J et al. **Music therapy** following suctioning: four case studies. Neonatal Netw 1995; 14(7):41-9.
41. Campos F, Waitzberg D, et al. Protective effects of **glutamine** enriched diets on acute actinic enteritis. Nutr Hosp 1996; 11(3):167-77
42. Carter C, Urbanowicz M, et al. Effects of a few food diet in **attention deficit disorder.** Arch Dis Child 1993; 69(5):564-8.

43. **Casby J, Holm M. The effect of music** on repetitive disruptive vocalizations of persons with dementia. Am J Occup Ther 1994; 48(10):883-9.
44. Cassileth B, Lusk E, et al. Survival and quality of life among patients receiving unproven as compared with conventional **cancer** therapy. , NEJM 1991; 324:1180-5.
45. Chandra R. **Nutrition and immunoregulation**. Significance for host resistance to tumors and infectious diseases in humans and rodents. J Nutr 1992; 122(3 Suppl):754-57.
46. Chandra R. **Nutrition and immuntiy**: an overview. J Nutr 1994; 124(8):1433S-35S.
47. Chang R. Functional properties of edible **mushrooms**. Nutr Rev 1996; 54(11 Pt 2):S91-3.
48. Chen Y, Shiao M, et al. Effect of **cordyceps sinensis** on the proliferation and differentiation of human leukemic U937 cells. Life Sci 1997; 60(25):2349-59.
49. Chlan L. Psychophysiologic responses of mechanically ventilated patients to **music**: a pilot study. Am J Crit Care 1995; 4(3):233-8
50. Chone B, Manidakis G. **Echinacin** test for the provocation of leukocytes in effective radiotherapy. Deutsch Med Wochenschr 1969; 94(27):1406-10.
51. Christenson G, Crow S. The characterization and treatment of **trichotillomania**. J Clin Psychiatry 1996; 57 Suppl 8:42-9
52. Chrubasik S, Kress W. Value of acupuncture in treatment of **migraine**. Anaesthesiol Reanim 1995; 20(6):150-2
53. Cocchi P. Antidepressant effect of **Vitamin C**. Pediatr 1980; 65(4):862-3.
54. Coeugniet E, Kuhnast R. Recurrent **candidiasis**: adjuvant immunotherapy with different formulations of Echinacin. Therapiewoche 1986; 36:3352-8.
55. Cohen MR, Isenberg D. Ultraviolet irradiation in systemic **lupus** erythematosus . . . Br J Rheumatol 1996; 35(10):1002-7
56. Constantinescu C., Melanin, **melatonin**, melanocyte-stimulating hormone . . . Med Hypotheses 1995; 45(5):455-8
57. Cott J. NCDEU update. Natural product formulations available in europe for **psychotropic** indications. Psychopharmacol Bull 1995; 31(4):745-51.
58. Cotterill J. Psychophysiological aspects of **eczema**. Semin Dermatol 1990; 9(3):216-9.
59. Dalgleish T, Rosen K, Marks M. **Rhythm and blues**: the theory and treatment . . . Br J Clin Psychol 1996; 35(Pt 2):163-82
60. de Lange de Klerk E, Blommers J, et al. Effect of **homeopathic** medicines on daily burden of symptoms . . . BMJ 1994; 309(6965):1329-32.
61. Der Marderosian A. Understanding **homeopathy**. J Am Pharm Assoc. 1996; Ns36(5):317-28.
62. DeSmet, PAGM et al. Adverse effects of **herbal drugs**. (Vol. I & II). New York: Springer-Verlag, 1993.
63. Devi P. **Withania** somnifera Dunal (Ashwagandha): potential plant source of a promising drug for cancer chemotherapy and radiosensitization. Indian J Exp Biol 1996; 34(10):927-32.

64. **Doll H, Brown S, et al. Pyridoxine (Vitamin B6) and the premenstrual** syndrome: a randomized crossover trial. J R Coll Gen Pract 1989; 39(326):364-8.
65. Donaldson R (ed). **Witch Hazel** works magic. Cortlandt Forum 1997; 10(3):112
66. dos Santos J. Supportive conservative therapies for **temporomandibular** disorders. Dent Clin North Am 1995; 39(2):459-77
67. Dowling E, Redondo D, et al. Effect of **Eleutherococcus** senticosus on submaximal and maximal exercise performance. Med Sci Sports Exerc 1996; 28(4):482-9.
68. Driskell J, et al. Effectiveness of pvridoxine hydrochloride treatment on **carpal tunnel** patients. Nutr Rep Int 1986; 34:1031-40.
69. Duke J. Handbook of Medicinal **Herbs**. Boca Raton, FL: CRC Press, 1985.
70. Duthie S. The effect of **dietary flavonoids** on DNA damage (strand breaks and oxidised pyrimdines) and growth in human cells. Mutat Res 1997; 390(1-2):141-51.
71. Dutkiewicz S. **Zinc and magnesium** serum levels in patients with . . . BPH . . . Mater Med Pol 1995; 27(1):15-7
72. Eastman C, Boulos Z, et al. **Light treatment** . . . shift work. J Biol Rhythms. 1995; 10(2):157-64
73. Edelstein S, Chisholm M. Management of intractable childhood **seizures** using the non-MCT oil ketogenic diet in 20 patients. J Am Diet Assoc 1996; 96(11):1181-2.
74. Elliott D. The effects of music and muscle relaxation on **patient anxiety** in a coronary care unit. Heart Lung 1994; 23(1):27-35
75. Ellis J, Folkers K. Clinical aspects of treatment of **carpal tunnel** syndrome with vitamin B6. Ann NY Acad Sci 1990; 585:302-20.
76. Elmer G, Surawicz C, McFarland L. **Biotherapeutic agents**. A neglected modality for the treatment and prevention of selected intestinal and vaginal infections. JAMA 1996; 276(1):29-30.
77. Elmore A. Biofeedback therapy in the treatment of **dental anxiety** and dental phobia. Dental Clinic North Amer 1988; 32(4):735-44.
78. Enstrom J, Kanim L, Klein M. **Vitamin C** intake and mortality among a sample of the United States population. Epidemiology 1992; 3:194-202.
79. Ernst E. **Complementary medicine: common misconceptions**. J R Soc Med 1995; 88:244-47.
80. Ernst E. Ginkgo biloba in treatment of **intermittent claudication**. Fortschr Med 1996; 114(8):85-7.
81. Ernst E. Risk-free **homeopathy**? Schweiz Med Wochenschr 1996; 126(40):1677-9
82. Ernst E. St. John's wort as **antidepressive** therapy. Fortschr Med 1995; 113(25):354-5.
83. Facts and Comparisons Publishing Group. The Review of **Natural Products**. St. Louis, MO: Facts and Comparisons, 1997. (Refers to latest monograph by subject).
84. Fahrion S. Self-regulation of **anxiety**. Bull Menninger Clin 1990; 54(2):217-31.
85. Fan C. Acupressure treatment for prevention of **postoperative nausea** and vomiting. Anesth Analg 1997; 84(4):821-5.
86. Farrugia G, Camilleri M, Whitehead W. Therapeutic strategies for

motility disorders. Gastroenterol Clin N Amer 1996; 25(1):225-46
87. Fontaine D. Nonpharmacologic management of **patient distress** during mechanical ventilation. Crit Care Clin 1994; 10(4):695-708.
88. Fontaine D. Nonpharmacologic management of patient distress during mechanical ventilation. Crit Care Clin 1994; 10(4):695-708.
89. Francis C, Houghton L. Use of **hypnotherapy** in gastrointestinal disorders. Eur J Gastroent Hepatol 1996; 8(6):525-9
90. Fraser G, Lindsted K, Beeson W. Effect of **risk factor** values on lifetime risk . . . Am J Epidem 1995; 142(7):746-58
91. Fraser G, Sabate J, Beeson WL. The application of results of some studies of California **Seventh-day Adventists** to the general population. Arch Int Med. 1993; 153:533-4.
92. Fraser G, Sabate J, et al. A possible protective effect of **nut consumption** on risk of coronary heart disease. Arch Int Med 1992; 152(7):1416-24
93. Frasure-Smith N, Lesperance F, et al. **Depression** following myocardial infarction. Impact on 6-month survival. JAMA 1993; 270(15):1819-25.
94. Freitag Pagliuca L. The **art** of communication in the fingertips. The blind person. Rev Lat Am Enfermagem 1996;4(suppl):127-37.
95. Fried R. Integrating **music** in breathing training and relaxation: background, rationale, and relevant elements. Biofeedback Self Regul 1990; 15(2):161-9.
96. Galsanov S, Tourova A, Klimenko E. Effect of **quercitrin** on structural changes in the large and small intestines in experimental enterocolitis. Biull Eksp Biol Med. 1976; 81(5):623-5.
97. Garg G, Nigam S, Ogle, C. The gastric antiulcer effects of the leaves of the **neem tree**. Planta Med. 1993; 59(3); 215-7.
98. Gattoni T, Parlavecchio L. **Theater art** as alternative psychotherapeutic treatment in an alcoholic patient. Minerva Psichiatr 1995; 36(1):51-6.
99. Ger E. **Mushrooms**: enjoying your medicine. Del Med J 1997; 69*3):149-51.
100. Gerhard U, Linnenbrink N, et al. Vegilance decreasing effects of 2 plant-derived **sedatives**. Schweiz Rundsch Med Prax 1996; 85(15):473-81.
101. Gibbs W, Wayt. Gaining on **fat**. Sci Amer 1996 (Aug):88-94
102. Gibson R, Gibson S, et al. **Homeopathic** therapy in rheumatoid arthritis: evaluation by double-blind clinical trial. Br J Clin Pharm. 1980; 9:453-459.
103. Gibson R, Gibson S, et al. Salicylates and homeopathy in **rheumatoid** arthritis: preliminary observations. Br J Cl Pharm. 1978; 6:391-395.
104. Gibson R. Content and bioavailability of **trace elements** in vegetarian diets. Am J Clin Nutr 1994; 59(suppl):1223s-32s.
105. Ginter E. Ascorbic acid in cholesterol metabolism and in detoxification of xenobiotic substances: problem of optimum **vitamin C** intake. Nutrition 1989; 5(6):369-74.
106. Giovannucci E. How is individual risk for **prostate cancer** assessed? Hematol Oncol Clin North Am 1996; 10(3):537-48
107. Glaister J. Projective drawings: helping adult **survivors of childhood abuse** recognize boundaries. J Psychosos Nurs Ment Health Serv. 1994;32(10):28-34.
108. Glaister J. Serial **self-portrait**: a technique to monitor changes in self

concept. Arch Psychiatr Nurs 1996; 10(5):311-8.
109. Good M. A comparison of the effects of jaw relaxation and **music** on postoperative pain. Nurs Res. 1995; 44(1)52-7.
110. Grant J, Veldee M, Buchwald D. Analysis of dietary intake and selected nutrient concentratins in patients with **chronic fatigue** syndrome. J Am Diet Assoc 1996; 96(4):383-6.
111. Grasha A, Homan M. Psychological size and distance in the relationships of **adult children of alcoholics** with their parents. Psychol Rep. 1995; 76(2):595-606.
112. Green J, Shellenberger R. The healing energy of **love**. Altern Ther Health Med 1996; 2(3):46-56
113. Groenewegen W, Knight D, Heptinstall S. Progress in the medicinal chemistry of the herb **feverfew**. Prog Med Chem 1992; 29:217-38.
114. Guy-Grand B, Crepaldi G, et al. International trial of long-term dexfenfluramine in **obesity**. The Lancet 1989; 11(8672):1142-1144
115. Hahnemann S. *Organon of Medicine.* (transl.) Blaine, Wash: Cooper Publishing, 1982.
116. Hall H, Minnes L, Olness K. The psychophysiology of voluntary **immunododulation**. Int J Neuro Sci 1993; 69(1-4):221-34
117. Hanser S, Thompson L. Effects of a **music** therapy strategy on depressed older adults. J Gerontol 1994; 49(6):265-9.
118. Harland B, Harden-Williams B. Is **vanadium** of human nutritional importance yet? J Am Diet Assoc 1994; 94(8):891-4.
119. Hashim S, Aboobaker V, et al. Modulatory effects of **essential oils** from spices on the formation of DNA adduct by aflatoxin B1 in vitro. Nutr Cancer 1994; 21(2):169-75.
120. Hatch G. **Asthma**, inhaled oxidants, and dietary antioxidants. Am J Clin Nutr. 1995; 61(3 Suppl):625S.
121. Havas S, Wozenski S, et al. Report of the New England Task Force on reducing **heart disease and stroke** risk. Pub Health Rep 1989;104(2):134-42
122. Heimendinger J. Community nutrition intervention strategies for **cancer risk** reduction. Cancer 1993; 72(3 Suppl):1019-23.
123. Hentschel C, Dressler S, Hahn E. Fumaria officinalis (**fumitory**)—clinical applications. Fortschr Med 1995; 113(19):291-2.
124. Herb Research Foundation. **Herb Safety Report**. Boulder, CO: Herb Research Foundation.
125. Herbert V, Subak-Sharpe G, (editors). *Total Nutrition: The Only Guide You'll ever need.* New York, NY: St. Martin's Press, 1995.
126. Hicks F. The role of **music** therapy in the care of the **newborn**. Nurs Times 1995; 91(38):31-3.
127. Hill N, Stam C, et al. A placebo controlled trial investigating the efficacy of a **homeopathic** after-bite gel . . . Eur J Clin Pharmacol 1995; 49(1-2):103-8.
128. Hirazumi A. Anticancer activity of Morinda citrtifolia (**noni**) on intraperitoneally implanted Lewis lung carcinoma in syngeneic mice. Proc West Pharmacol Soc. 1994; 37:145-6.
129. Hirazumi A. Immunomodulation contributes to the anticancer activity of morinda citrifolia (**noni**) fruit juice. Proc West Pharmacol Soc 1996; 39:7-9.
130. Hobbs C. The **Echinacea** Handbook. Portland, OR: Eclectic Medical Publications, 1989.
131. Hochstrasser B, Mattmann P. **Homeopathy** and conventional

medicine... Schweiz Med Wochenschr Suppl 1994;62:28-35
132. Hornig-Rohan M, Wolkowitz O, Amsterdam J. Novel strategies for **treatment-resistant depression**. Psychiatr Clin N Am 1996; 19(2):387-405
133. Horrobin DF. Essential fatty acid and prostaglandin metabolism in **Sjogren's** syndrome, **systemic sclerosis** and **rheumatoid arthritis**. Scand J Rheumatol Suppl 1986; 61:242-5.
134. Hoyer S. Possibilities and limits of therapy of **cognition disorders** in the elderly. Z Gerontol Geriatr 1995; 28(6):457-62.
135. Hunt CD. The biochemical effects of physiologic amounts of dietary **boron** in animal nutrition models. Environ Health Perspect 1994; 102 Suppl 7:35-43.
136. Hunt J. Position of the American Dietetic Association: **vitamin and mineral** supplementation. J Am Diet Assoc 1996;96(1):73ff.
137. Hutt G. **Hypnotherapy** and acute pain control. Br J Theatre Nurs 1996; 5(12):18-21
138. Innis S. **Essential fatty acid** requirements in human nutrition. Can J Pharm 1993; 71(9):699-706.
139. Inselmann U. Treatment of psychotic patients with **music** therapy. Z Klin Psychol Psychopathol Psychother 1995; 43(3):249-60.
140. Jacobs J, Jimenez L, et al. **Homeopathic** treatment of acute childhood diarrhea with homeopathic medicine: a randomized clinical trial in Nicaragua. Pediatrics 1994; 93:719-725.
141. Janelle K, Barr S. Nutrient intakes and eating behavior scores of **vegetarian** and nonvegetarian women. J Am Diet Assoc 1995; 95(2):180-6, 189.
142. Jonas W, Jacobs J. *Healing with Homeopathy: The Complete Guide.* New York, NY: Warner Books, Inc., 1996.
143. Jossa F, Mancini M. The **Mediterranean diet** in the prevention of arteriosclerosis. Recenti Prog Med. 1996; 87(4):175-81.
144. Kaminski J, Hall W. The effect of soothing **music** on **neonatal** behavioral states in the hospital newborn nursery. Neonatal Netw 1996; 15(1)45-54.
145. Kanter M, Williams M. Antioxidants, carnitine, and choline as putative **ergogenic** aids. Int J Sport Nutr 1995; 5 Suppl: S120-31
146. Katiyar S. Protective effects of **silymarin** against photocarcinogenesis in a mouse skin model. J Natl Cancer Inst 1997; 89(8):556-66.
147. Kerscher M, Korting H. Treatment of atopic **eczema** with evening primrose oil: rationale and clinical results. Clin Investig 1992; 70(2):167-71.
148. Kim I, Williamson D, et al. **Vitamin and mineral** supplement use and mortality in a US cohort. Am J Public Health 1993; 83:546-550.
149. Kimmick G, Bell R, Bostick R. **Vitamin E** and breast cancer: a review. Nutr Cancer 1997; 27(2):109-17.
150. Kleijnen J, Knipschild P, Ter Riet G. Clinical trials of **homeopathy**. Br Med J 1991; 302:316-23.
151. Klein S, Winkelstein M. Enhancing pediatric health care with **music**. J Pediatr Health Care 1996; 10(2):74-81.
152. Klein T. **Stress and infections**. J Fla Med Assoc. 1993; 80(6): 409-11
153. Knight DW. **Feverfew**: chemistry and biological activity. Nat Prod Rep. 1995; 12(3):271-6.
154. Kraft M, Martin R. Chronobiology and chronotherapy **in medicine**

Dis Mon 1995 Aug; 41(8):501-75.
155. Krishnaswamy K, Polasa K. **Diet, nutrition & cancer**—the Indian scenario. Indian J Med Res 1995; 102:200-9.
156. Krishnaswamy K. **Indian** functional **foods**: role in prevention of cancer. Nutr Rev 1996; 54(11 Pt 2):S127-31.
157. Krummel D, Seligson F, Guthrie H. **Hyperactivity**: is candy causal? Crit Rev Food Sci Nutr 1996; 36(1-2):31-47.
158. Kubo K, Nauba H. The effect of **maitake mushrooms** on liver and serum lipids. Altern Ther Health Med 1996; 2(5):62-6.
159. Kubo K. The effect of maitake mushrooms on liver and serum lipids. Altern Ther Health Med 1996; 2(5):62-6.
160. Kudrin A. Current concept of scientific pharmacotherapy. Role of **nutrition** in the regulation of body's vital activity and homeostasis. Vestn Ross Akad Med Nauk 1996; 12:20-23.
161. Kuo Y. **Cordyceps sinensis** as an immunomodulatory agent. Am J Chin Med 1996; 24(2):111-25.
162. Kuo Y. Growth inhibitors against tumor cells in **Cordyceps sinensis** other than cordycepin and polysaccharides. Cancer Invest 1994; 12(6):611-5.
163. Kupfer DJ, Reynolds III CF. Management of **Insomnia**. New Engl J Med 1997; 336 (5):341-6.
164. Lane M, Graham-Pole J. Development of an **art** program on a bone marrow transplant unit. Cancer Nurs 1994;17(3):185-92.
165. Lehna C. **Children's** descriptions of their feelings and what they found helpful during **bereavement**. Am J Hosp Palliat Care 1995; 12(5):24-30.
166. Lehrer P. **Stress** management techniques: are they all equivalent, or do they have specific effects? Biofeedback Self Regul 1994; 19(4):353-401.
167. Levenson D, Bockman R. A review of **calcium** preparations. Nutr Rev 1994; 52(7):221-32. (note correction 52(10):364).
168. Levin JS. How **prayer** heals: a theoretical model. Altern Ther Health Med 1996; 2(1):66-73
169. Levine G, Balady G. The benefits and risks of **exercise** training: the exercise prescription. Adv Intern Med 1993; 38:57-79
170. Lewis TA, Solomon GD. Advances in **migraine** management. Cleve Clin J Med 1995; 62(3):148-55
171. Lin X. Therapeutic effect of **Ganoderma** applonatum (GA) on chronic **hepatitis B**. Chung Hua Nei Ko Tsa Chih 1988; 27(10):618-20.
172. Lin Y. Acupuncture treatment for **insomnia** and acupuncture analgesia. Psychiatry Clin Neurosci 1995; 49(2):119-20
173. Lokken P, Straumsheim P, et al. Effect of **homeopathy** on pain and other events after acute trauma . . . BMJ 1995; 310(6992):1439-42.
174. Lubar J, Swartwood M, et al. Evaluation of the effectiveness of EEG neurofeedback training for **ADHD** in a clinical setting as a measured by changes in T.O.V.A. scores, behavioral ratings, and WISC-R performance. Biofeedback Self Regul 1995; 201(1):83-99.
175. Lukaski H, Bolonchuk W, et al. **Chromium** supplementation and resistance training: effects on body composition, strength, and trace element status of men. Am J Clin Nutr 1996; 63(6):954-65.
176. Lukaski H. **Micronutrients** (magnesium, zinc and copper): are mineral supplements needed for athletes? Int J Sport Nutr 1995 Jun; 5 Suppl: s74-83.

177. Lund D, Hill R, et al. Video respite: an innovative resource for family, professional caregivers, and persons with dementia. Gerontologist. 1995; 35(5):683-7.
178. Maberly G, Trowbridge F, et al. Programs against **micronutrient** malnutriton . . . Annu Rev Publ Health 1994; 15:277-301.
179. MacLean L, Rhode B, et al. Results of the surgical treatment of **obesity**. Am J Surg. 1993; 165(1):155-62.
180. Mallett J. Use of **humor** and laughter in patient care. Br J Nurs 1993; 2(3):172-5
181. Mares-Perlman J, Brady W, et al. Diet and nuclear **lens opacities**. Am J Epidemiol 1995; 141(4):322-34.
182. Maslova L, Lishmanov, I, Maslov L. **Cardioprotective** effects of adaptogens of plant origin. Biull Eksp Biol Med 1993; 115(3):269-71.
183. Massad S, Shier N et al. High school **athletes** and **nutritional** supplements: a study of knowledge and use. Int J Sport Nutr 1995; 5(3):232-45.
184. Matheson I. Infantile **colic**—what will help? Tidsskr Nor Laegeforen 1995; 115(19):2386-9
185. Maughan R. **Creatine** supplementation and exercise performance. Int J Sport Nutr 1995; 5(2):94-101
186. McCarty M. Homologous physiological effects of phenformin and **chromium** picolinate. Med Hypotheses 1993; 41(4):316-24
187. McGinnis J, Foege W. **Actual causes of death in the United States**. JAMA 1993; 270(18):2207-2212
188. Meydani S, Meydani M, et al. **Vitamin E** supplementation and in vivo immune response in healthy elderly subjects. A randomized controlled trial. JAMA 1997; 277(17):1380-6.
189. Meyers D, Maloley P, Weeks D. Safety of **antioxidant** vitamins. Arch Intern Med. 1996; 156(9):925-35.
190. Milewicz A, Gejdel E, et al. Vitex agnus castus extract in the treatment of **luteal phase** defects due to latent hyperprolactinemia. Results of a randomized placebo-controlled double-blind study. Arzneimittelforschung 1993; 43(7):752-6.
191. Miller K, Billings D. **Playing** to grow: a primary mental health intervention with Guatamalan refugee children. Am J Orthopsychiatry 1994;64(3):346-56.
192. Mills P, Beeson WL, et al. **Cancer** incidence among California Seventh-day Adventists, 1976-1982. Am J Clin Nutr 1994; 59(suppl):1136s-42s.
193. Mishra A, Singh N, Sharma V. Use of **neem oil** as a mosquito repellent in tribal villages of manla district, madhya pradesh. Indian J Malariol 1995; 32(3):99-103.
194. Mital B, Garg S. Anticarcinogenic, hypocholesterolemic and antagonistic activities of Lactobacillus **acidophilus**. Crit Rev Microbiol 1995; 21(3):175-214.

References

196. Moore J. An assessment of **boric acid** and borax using the IEHR evaluative process for assessing human developmental and reproductive toxicity of agents. Reprod Toxicol 1997; 11(1):123-60.
197. Moriguchi S, Miwa H, Kishino Y. **Glutamine** supplementation prevents the decrease of mitogen response . . . J Nutr Sci Vitam 1995;41(1):115-25
198. Morley J. **Nutrition and the older female**: a review. J Am Col Nutr 1993; 12(4):337-43.
199. Mornhinweg G, Voignier R. **Music** for sleep disturbance in the elderly. J Holist Nurs 1995; 13(3):248-54.
200. Mulloney SS, Wells-Federman C. Therapeutic **touch**: a healing modality. J Cardiovasc Nurs 1996; 10(3):27-49
201. Murphy J, Heptinstall S, Mitchell J. Randomised double-blind placebo-controlled trial of **feverfew** in migraine prevention. Lancet 1988; 2(8604):189-92.
202. Mynchenberg T, Cungan J. A relaxation protocol to reduce patient **anxiety**. Dimens Crit Care Nurs 1995; 14(2):78-85.
203. Nakata S, Sato J, et al. Epidemiological characteristics of **prostate** cancer in Gunma Prefecture, Japan. Int J Urol 1995; 2(3):191-7
204. Nanba H. Activity of **maitake** D-fraction to inhibit carcinogenesis and metastasis. Ann N Y Acad Sci 1995; 768:243-5.
205. Neeleman J, Persaud R. Why do psychiatrists neglect **religion**? Br J Med Psychol 1995; 68(Pt 2):169-78
206. Cohen S, Tyrrell DA, Smith AP. Psychological **stress** and susceptibility to the **common cold**. NEJM 1991; 325(9):606-12.
207. Nestle M. **Fruits** and **vegetables**: protective or just fellow travelers? Nutr Rev 1996; 54(8):255-7.
208. Newsweek. The medical bottom line. Feb. 3, 1997, p. 23
209. Nicholas J. Physical modalities in **rheumatological** rehabilitation. Arch Phys Med Rehabil 1994; 75:994-1001.
210. Nielsen F. How should dietary guidance be given for **mineral** elements with beneficial actions or suspected of being essential? J Nutr 1996; 126 (9 Suppl):2377S-85S.
211. Nieman D, Ahle J, eta l. Indomethacin does not alter natural killer cell response to 2.5 h of running. J Appl Physiol 1995; 79(3):748-55
212. Nieman D, Cook V, eta l. Moderate **exercise** training and natural killer cell cytotoxic activity . . . Int J Sports Med 1995; 16(5):334-7
213. Nieman D, Henson D. Role of endurance **exercise** in immune senescence. Med Sci Sports Exerc 1994; 26(2):172-81
214. Nieman D. Exercise, infection, and **immunity**. Int J Sports Med. 1994 Oct; 15 Suppl 3:S131-41
215. Nieman D. Upper respiratory tract **infections** and **exercise**. Thorax 1995; 50(12):1229-31
216. Nieman, D. **Fitness and Sports Medicine**: An Introduction. Palo Alto, CA: Bull Publishing Company, 1990.
217. NIH Consensus Conference. Gastrointestinal surgery for severe **obesity** . . . Am J Clin Nutr 1992; 55 (2 Suppl):615S-619S.
218. NIH Technology Assessment Panel on Integration of **Behavioral** and Relaxation . . . JAMA 1996; 276(4):313-8
219. O'Callaghan C. Pain, **music** creativity and music therapy in palliative care. Am J Hosp Palliat Care 1996; 13(2):43-9.
220. O'Connor P (ed). Red Meat-**Psoriasis** link. Cortlandt Forum 1997; 10(3):100

221. Ofek I, Goldhar J, Sharon N. Anti-Escherichia coli adhesin activity of **cranberry** and **blueberry** juices. Adv Exp Med Biol 1996; (408):179-83.
222. Ornish D, Brown S, et al. Can lifestyle changes reverse coronary heart disease? **The lifestyle heart trial**. Lancet 1990; 336:129-33.
223. Ornish D, Brown S, et al. Can lifestyle changes reverse coronary heart disease? The Lifestyle Heart Trial. Lancet 1990; 336(8708):129-33.
224. Ornish D. Lifestyle changes and heart disease. Lancet 1990; 336(8717):741-2.
225. Ornish D. **Reversing heart disease** through diet, exercise, and stress management: an interview with Dean Ornish. J Am Diet Assoc 1991; 91(2):162-5.
226. Parry G, Bredesen D. Sensory neuropathy with low-dose **pyridoxine**. Neurology 1985; 35:1466-8.
227. Pattrick M, Heptinstall S, Doherty M. **Feverfew** in rheumatoid arthritis: a double blind, placebo controlled study. Ann Rheum Dis 1989; 48(7):547-9.
228. Pedersen B, Bruunsgaard H. How physical **exercise** influences the establishment of infections. Sports Med 1995; 19(6):393-400
229. Peloquin S. **Art**: an occupation with promise for developing empathy. Am J Occup Ther 1996; 50(8):655-61.
230. Perharic L, Shaw D, et al. **Toxicological** problems resulting from exposure to traditional remedies and food supplements. Drug Saf 1994; 11(4):284-94
231. Perry P, Dean B, Krenzelok E. **Cinnamon** oil abuse by adolescents. Vet Hum Toxicol. 1990; 32(2):162-4.
232. Peters C, Lotzerich H, et al. Influence of a moderate **exercise** training on natural killer cytotoxicity . . . Anticancer Res 1994; 14(3A):1033-6
233. Peters E, Goetzsche J, et al. **Vitamin C** supplementation reduces the incidence of postrace symptoms of upper-respiratory-tract infection in ultramarathon runners. Am J Clin Nutr 1993; 57(2):170-4.
234. Peterson J. **Acupuncture** in the 1990s . . .Arch Fam Med 1996; 5:237-41.
235. Pohl P. Therapy of radiation-induced leukopenia by **esberitox**. Med Klin 1969; 64:1546-7.
236. Polyp Prevention Study Group. A clinical trial of **antioxidant** vitamins to prevent colorectal adenoma. N Engl J Med. 1994; 331:141-7.
237. Potter J, Steinmetz K. Vegetables, fruit and **phytoestrogens** as preventive agents. IARC Sci Publ 1996;(139):61-90. (A review with 205 references).
238. Pratt L, Ford D, et al. **Depression**, psychotropic medication, and risk of **myocardial infarction**. Prospective data from the Baltimore ECA follow up. Circulation. 1996; 94(12):3123-9.
239. Prentice A, Bates C. Adequacy of dietary **mineral** supply for human bone growth and mineralisation. Eur J Clin Nutr 1994; 48 Suppl 1:s161-77.
240. Purdie H, Baldwin S. Models of **music** therapy intervention in stroke rehabilitation. Int. J Rehabil Res 1995; 18(4):341-50.
241. Quale J, Landman D, et al. In vitro activity of Cinnamomum zeylanicum against azole resistant and sensitive Candida species and a pilot study of **cinnamon** for oral candidiasis. Am J Chin Med 1996; 24(2):103-9.

242. Radtke P. **Art** and rehabilitation. Rehabilitation (Stuttg) 1994;33(2):61-3.
243. Ragneskog H, et al. Influence of dinner **music** on food intake and symptoms common in dementia. Scand J Caring Sci 1996; 10(1):11f.
244. Rapola J, Virtamo J, et al. Randomised trial of **alpha-tocopherol** and **beta-carotene** supplements on incidence of major coronary events in men with previous myocardial infarction. Lancet 1997; 349(9067):1715-20.
245. Rautalahti M, Huttunen J. **Antioxidants** and carcinogenesis. Ann Med 1994; 26(6):435-41
246. Reichart P. Oral cancer and precancer related to **betel** and miang chewing in Thailand: a review. J Oral Pathol Med 1995; 24(6):241-3.
247. Richmond C. A **homeopathic** fatality. Can Med Assoc J. 1992; 147(1):97-8.
248. Rimm E, Stampfer M, eta l. **Vitamin E** consumption and the risk of coronary disease in men. N Engl J Med. 1993; 328:1450-56.
249. Rosenblatt M, Mindel J. Spontaneous hyphema associated with ingestion of **Ginkgo biloba** extract. NEJM 1997; 336(15):1108.
250. Rowe KS, Rowe KJ. Synthetic **food coloring** and behavior: a dose response effect in a double-blind, placebo-controlled, repeated-measure study. J Pediatr 1994; 125(5 Pt 1):691-8.
251. Sabo C, Michael S. The influence of personal message with **music** on anxiety and side effects associated with chemotherapy. Cancer Nurs 1996; 19(4):283-9.
252. Sagar P. Surgical treatment of morbid **obesity**. Br J Surg 1995; 82(6):732-9.
253. Salmeron J, Manson J, et al. **Dietary fiber**, glycemic load, and risk of non-insulin-dependent diabetes mellitus in women. JAMA 1997; 277(6):472-7
254. Sander D, Scholz C, et al. Plexus neuropathy following vaccination . . . Neurol Res 1995; 17(4):316-9
255. Sandyk R. Premenstrual exacerbation of symptoms in **multiple sclerosis** . . . Int J Neurosci 1995; 83(3-4):187-98
256. Saper B. The therapeutic use of **humor** for psychiatric disturbances of adolescents and adults. Psychiat Q 1990; 61(4):261-72
257. Schedlowski M, Schmidt R. **Stress** and the immune system. Naturwissenschaften 1996; 83(5):214-20
258. Schoneberger D. The influence of immune-stimulating effects of pressed juice from **echinacea** purpurea on the course and severity of colds. Forum Immunologie 1992; 8:2-12.
259. Schroeder-Sheker T. **Music** for the dying: a personal account of the new field of music thanatology. J Holist Nurs 1994; 12(1):83-99.
260. Schut H, de Keijser J, et al. Cross-modality **grief** therapy: description and assessment. . . J Clin Psychol 1996; 52(3):357-65.
261. Schwartz J, Weiss S. Relationship between dietary **vitamin C** intake and **pulmonary** functions in the First National Health and Nutrition Examination Survey (NHANES I). Am J Clin Nutr 1994; 59(1):110-114.
262. Scofield M, Martin W. Development of the AT&T **Health Audit** for measuring organizational health. Occup Med 1990; 5(4):755-70
263. Seaborn C, Nielsen F. Effects of **germanium** and **silicon** on bone mineralization. Biol Trace Elem Res 1994; 42(2):151-64.

264. Shakila R, Vasundhara T, Rao D. Inhibitory effect of **spices** on in vitro histamine production and histidine decarboxylase activity of Morganella morganii and on the biogenic amine formation in mackerel stored at 30 degrees C. Z Lebensm Unters Forsch 1996; 203(1):71-6.
265. Shaw CR. The perimenopausal **hot flash**: epidemiology, physiology, and treatment. Nurse Pract 1997; 22(3):55-66.
266. Shek P, Sabiston B, et al. Strenuous **exercise** and immunological changes . . . Int J Sports Med 1995; 16(7):466-74
267. Shelton H. **Natural Hygiene**: the Pristine Way of Life. 1995 ed. Introduction by Ronald Cridland
268. Shephard R, Shek P. Cancer, immune function, and **physical activity**. Can J Appl Physiol 1995; 20(1):1-25
269. Shephard R. A critical analysis of **work-site fitness** programs and their postulated economic benefits. Med Sci Sports Exerc 1992; 24(3):354-70
270. Shinkai S, Kohno H, et al. **Physical activity** and immune senescence in men. Med Sci Sports Exerc 1995; 27(11):1516-26
271. Simms RW. Controlled trials of therapy in **fibromyalgia** syndrome. Baillieres Clin Rhematol 1994; 8(4):917-34
272. Singh A, Failla M, Deuster P. **Exercise**-induced changes in immunce function: effects of zinc . . . J Appl Physiol 1994; 76(6):2298-303
273. Singh H, Srivastava M, et al. **Cinnamon** bark oil, a potent fungitoxicant against fungi causing respiratory tract mycoses. Allergy 1995; 50(12):995-9.
274. Skowron J, Tyszkiewicz M. **Art** therapy as an assisting psychotherapeutic method for adolescents. Psychiatr Pol 1996; 30(2):247-54.
275. Smith P, Maclennan K, Darlington C. The neuroprotective properties of the **Ginkgo biloba** leaf: a review of the possible relationship to platelet-activating factor (PAF). J Ethnopharmacol 1996; 50(3):131-9.
276. Smith RS. The cytokine theory of **headache**. Med Hypotheses 1992; 39(2):168-74.
277. Smith SM, McDonald A, Natow A, Heslin J. ***Complete Book of Vitamins & Minerals.*** Lincolnwood, ILL: Publications International, Ltd. 1996.
278. Soffa V. Alternatives to hormone replacement for **menopause**. Altern Ther Health Med 1996; 2(2):34-9
279. Spigelblatt L. Alternative Medicine: should it be used by **children**? Curr Probl Pediatr 1995; 25:180-8.
280. Stampfer M, Hemekens C, et al. **Vitamin E** consumption and the risk of coronary disease in women. N Eng J Med 1993; 328:1444-9.
281. Standley J, Hanser S. **Music** therapy research and applications in pediatric oncology treatment. J Pediatr Oncol Nurs 1995; 12(1):3-10.
282. Standley J, Moore R. Therapeutic effects of **music** and mother's voice on **premature infants**. Pediatr Nurs 1995; 21(6):509-12, 574.
283. Stearns D, Belbruno J, Wetterhahn K. A prediction of **chromium** (III) accumulation in humans from chromium dietary supplements. FASEB J 1995; 9(15):1650-7
284. Steerenberg P. The effect of oral **quercetin** on UVB-induced tumor growth and local immunosuppression in SKH-1. Cancer Lett 1997; 114(1-2):187-9.
285. Sterritt P, Pokorny M. **Art** activities for patients with **Alzheimer's** and related disorders. Geriatr Nurs 1994;15(3):155-9.

286. Stix G. Village pharmacy. **The neem** tree yields products from pesticides to soap. Sci Am 1992; 266(5):132.
287. Stransky M, et al. Treatment of **carpal tunnel** syndrome with vitamin B6: a double blind study. South Med J. 1989; 82(7):841-2.
288. Strivastava K. Extracts from two frequently consumed spices—**cumin** (Cuminum cyminum) and **turmeric** (Curcuma longa)—inhibit platelet aggregation and alter eicosanoid biosynthesis in human blood platelets. Prostaglandins Leukot Essent Fatty Acids 1989; 37(1):57-64.
289. Surh Y, Lee S. **Capsaicin** in hot chili pepper: carcinogen, co-carcinogen or anticarcinogen? Food Chem Toxicol 1996; 34(3):313-6.
290. Talwar G, Raghuvanshi P, et al. Plant immunomodulators for termination of unwanted pregnancy and for **contraception** and reproductive health. Immunol Cell Biol 1997; 75(2):190-2.
291. Tan G, Schneider S. **Attention-deficit** hyperactivity disorder. Pharmacotherapy and beyond. Postgrad Med 1997; 101(5):201-4.
292. Tanaka S, Yoon Y, et al. Antiulcerogenic compounds isolated from Chinese **cinnamon**. Planta Med 1989; 55(3):245-8.
293. Tang W, Yao X, Zheng Z. Rehabilitative effect of **music** therapy for residual schizophrenia. Br J Psychiatry Suppl 1994; 24:38-44.
294. Tantaoui-Elaraki A, Beraoud L. Inhibition of growth and **aflatoxin** production in Aspergillus parasiticus by essential oils of selected plant materials. J Environ Pathol Toxicol Oncol 1994; 13(1):67-72.
295. Terman M, Lewy A, et al. **Light** treatment for sleep disorders: consensus report. IV . . . J Biol Rhythms 1995; 10(2):135-47
296. The Medical Letter. Dexfenfluramine for **obesity** 1996; 38(979):64-5.
297. Tribble D, Frank E. Dietary **antioxidants**, cancer and atherosclerotic heart disease. West J Med 1994; 161(6):605-12
298. Tsi D, Tan B. Effects of **celery** extract and 3-N-butylphthalide on lipid levels in genetically hypercholesterolaemic (RICO) rats. Clin Exp Pharmacol Physiol 1996; 23(3):214-7.
299. Turley J, Fu T, et al. **Vitamin E** succinate induces Fas-mediated apoptosis in estrogen receptor-negative human breast cancer cells. Cancer Res 1997; 57(5):881-90.
300. Tyler V. **Herbs of Choice**: *The therapeutic use of phytomedicinals.* Binghamton, NY: The Hawthorn Press, Inc., 1994.
301. Tyler V. **The Honest Herbal**: *a sensible guide to the use of herbs and related remedies, third edition.* Binghamton, NY: The Hawthorn Press, Inc., 1993.
302. Tyszkiewicz M. **Art** therapy as a stimulation in the process of social adjustment of schizophrenia patients. Psychiatr Pol 1994;28(2):183-90.
303. Ubbink J, Becker P, Vermaak W. Will an increased dietary **folate** intake reduce the incidence of cardiovascular disease? Nut Rev 1996;54(7):213-6
304. Uhari M, Kontiokari T, et al. **Xylitol** chewing gum in prevention of acute **otitis media**: double blind randomised trial. BMJ 1996; 313(7066):1180-4.
305. Uthus E, Seaborn C. Deliberations and evaluations of the approaches, endpoints and paradigms for dietary recommendations of the other **trace elements**. J Nutr 1996; 126 (9 Suppl): 2452S-9S).
306. Vazquez F, Suarez M, Perez A. **Medicinal plants** used in the Barros Area, Badajoz Province, Spain. J Ethnopharmacol 1997; 55(2):81-5.

307. Velraeds MM, van der Mei H, et al. Inhibition of initial adhesion of uropathogenic Enterococcus faecalis to solid substrata by an adsorbed biosurfactant layer from **Lactobacillus acidophilus**. Urology 1997; 49(5):790-4.
308. Velussi M. Long term (12 months) treatment with an anti-oxidant drug (**silymarin**) is effective on hyperinsulinemia, exogenous insulin need and malondialdehyde levels in cirrhotic **diabetic** patients. J Hepatol 1997; 26(4):871-9.
309. Vickers A. Can **acupuncture** have specific effects on health? . . . J R Soc Med 1996; 89:303-311.
310. Viru A, Smirnova T. Health promotion and **exercise** training. Sports Med 1995; 19(2):123-36
311. Walach H. Is **homeopathy** accessible to research? Schweiz Rundsch Med Prax 1994; 83(51-52):1439-47
312. Walsh S, Hardin S. An **art** future image intervention to enhance identity and self-efficacy in adolescents. J Child Adolesc Psychiatr Nurs 1994; 7(3):24-34.
313. Weintraub M, Sundaresan P, et al. Long-term **weight control** study. IV (weeks 156-190) . . . Clin Pharmacol Ther 1992; 51(5):608-14.
314. Weintraub M. Long-term weight control . . . Clin Pharmacol Ther 1992; 51(5):581-5.
315. Wenneberg S, Schneider R, et al. **Anger** expression correlates with platelet aggregation. Behav Med 1997; 22(4):174-7.
316. Werbach M, Murray M. *Botanical Influences on Illness: A sourcebook of clinical research.* Tarzana, CA: Third Line Press, 1994.
317. Werbach, M. *Nutritional Influences on Illness, A Sourcebook of Clinical Research, second edition.* Tarzana, CA: Third Line Press, 1996.
318. White P. Are nonpharmacologic techniques useful alternatives to **antiemetic** drugs for the prevention of nausea and vomiting? Anesth Analg 1997; 84(4):712-4.
319. Whiting S. Safety of some **calcium** supplements questioned. Nutr Rev 1994; 52(3):95-7
320. Wimpory D, Chadwick P et al. Brief report: **musical** interaction therapy for children with **autism** . . . J Austism Dev Disord 1995; 25(5):541-52.
321. Winter M, Paskin S, Baker T. **Music** reduces stress and anxiety of patients in the surgical holding area. J Post Anesth Nurs. 1994; 9(6):340-3.
322. Wolraich M, Lindgren S, et al. Effects of diets high in **sucrose** or **aspartame** on the behavior and cognitive performance of children. N Engl J Med 1994; 330(5):301-7.
323. Wootan M, Liebman B, Rosofsky W. **Trans**: the phantom fat. Nutrition Action Health Letter 1996; 23(7):1, 10-13
324. Wooten P. **Humor**: an antidote for stress. Holist Nurs Pract 1996; 10(2):49-56
325. Woteki C. Applications of **antioxidants** in physiologically functional foods. Crit Rev Food Sci Nutr 1995; 35(1-2):143-7
326. Wright E, Schiffman E. Treatment alternatives for patients with **masticatory** myofascial **pain**. J Am Dent Assoc 1995; 126(7):1030-9
327. Wu T. Lead poisoning caused by contaminated **Cordyceps**, a Chinese herbal medicine: two case reports. Sci Total Environ 1996; 182(1-3):193-5.

328. Yamada K, Miura T, et al. Effect of inhalation of **chamomile** oil vapour on plasma ACTH level in ovariectomized-rat under restriction stress. Biol Pharm Bull 1996; 19(9):1244-6.
329. Yamamoto M, Uemura T, et al. Serum HDL-cholesterol-increasing and fatty liver-improving action of panax **ginseng** in high cholesterol diet-fed rats with clinical effect on hyperlipidemia in man. Am J Clin Med. 1983; 11:96-101.
330. Youngston R. Randomized trial of **homeopathic** arnica [letter] J R Soc Med 1997; 90(4):239-40.
331. Younos C, Rolland A, et al. Analgesic and behavioral effects of **Morinda** citrifolia. Planta Med 1990; 56(5):430-4.
332. Z'Brun A. **Ginkgo**—myth and reality. Schweiz Rundsch Med Prax 1995; 84(1):1-6.
333. Zaichkowsky L. **Biofeedback** applications in exercise and athletic performance. Exerc Sport Sci Rev. 16. 1988; 381-421.
334. Zaitsev A, Sorokina E, et al. **Cranberries**: chemical composition, nutritional and medicinal properties. Vopr Pitan 1997; (2):38-40.
335. Zaitsev A. **Cranberries**: chemical compostition, nutritional and medicinal properties. Vopr Pitan 1997; 2:38-40.
336. Zhang Z, Su C, Chen D. Comparison of **bacteriostatic** ability of oleum of Perilla frutescens (L.) Britt., Cinnamomum cassia Presl and Nipagin A. Chung Kuo Chung Yao Tsa Chinh. 1990; 15(2):95-7, 126-7.
337. Ziba M. Preliminary laboratory trial of **Neem** on anopheles and culex larvae in Zambia. Cent Afr J Med 1995; 41(4):137-8.
338. Zwicky J, Hafner A, Barrett S, Jarvis W. *Reader's Guide to Alternative Health Methods.* American Medical Association: 1993.
339. Zyss T, Krawczyk A. **Magnetic** brain stimulation in treatment of **depression** . . . Psychiatr Pol 1996; 30(4):611-28
340. reference deleted
341. Morice A. Adulterated "**homeopathic**" cure for asthma. Lancet 1986; 1(8485):862-3.
342. Reilly, D. Data presented at Alternative Medicine symposium (Harvard Medical School, Dept. of CME) March 9, 1997 (Boston)
343. Labrecque M. **Homeopathic** treatment of plantar warts. Can Med Assoc J. 1992; 146(10):1749-53.
344. Zanolla R, Monzeglio C, et al. Evaluation of the results of three different methods of postmastectomy **lymphedema** treatment. J Surg Oncol 1984; 26(3):210-13.
345. Becker H. Quantitative assessment of postoperative breast **massage**. Plast Reconstr Surg 1990; 86(2):355-6.
346. Field T, Grizzle N, et al. **Massage** and relaxation therapies' effects on depressed adolescent mothers. Adolescence 1996; 31(124):903-11.
347. Ironson G, Field T, et al. **Massage** therapy is associated with enhancement of the immune system's cytotoxic capacity. Int J Neurosci 1996: 84(1-4):205-17.
348. Ames BN, Gold LS. The **causes and prevention of cancer**: gaining perspective. Environ Health Perspect 1997; 105 (Suppl. 4): 865-73.
349. Field T, Quintino O, et al. **Job stress** reduction therapies. Altern Ther Health Med. 1997; 3(4):54-6.
350. see ref. 401.
351. White AR, Rampes H. Acupuncture in smoking cessation. In: Lancaster T, Silagy C (eds) Tobacco Addiction Module of The

Cochrane Database of Systematic Reviews, [updated 02 December 1996]. Oxford: Update Software; 1997.
352. Cohen S, Line S, et al. Chronic social stress, social stress, and susceptibility to **upper respiratory infections** in nonhuman primates. Psychosom Med. 1997; 59(3):213-21. See also ref. 387 and 389.
353. Labott S, Ahleman S, et al. The physiological and psychological effects of the expression and inhibition of **emotion**. Behav Med 1990; 16(4):182-9.
354. Pennebaker J, et al. Putting **stress** into words: health, linguistic, and therapeutic implications. Behav Res Ther 1993; 31(6):539-48.
355. Stone A, Neale J, et al. Daily events are associated with a secretory **immune** response to an oral antigen in men. Health Psychol 1994; 13(5):440-6.
356. Keicolt-Glaser J, et al. Slowing of **wound healing** by psychological stress. Lancet. 1995; 346(8984):1194-6.
357. ref. deleted
358. Keicolt-Glaser J, Glaser R, et al. **Marital conflict** in older adults: endocrinological and immunological correlates. Psychosom Med. 1997; 59(4):339-49.
359. ref. deleted
360. Palakanis K, DeNobile J, et al. Effect of **music** therapy on state anxiety in patients undergoing flexible sigmoidoscopy. Dis Colon Rectum 1994; 37(5):478-81.
361. Easter A. The state of research on the effects of **therapeutic touch**. J Holist Nurs 1997; 15(2):158-75.
362. Glickman R, Burns J. If **therapeutic touch** works, prove it! RN 1996; 59(12):76.
363. Rackett S, Rothe M, Grant-Kels J. **Diet and dermatology**... J Am Acad Derm. 1993; 29(3):447-61.
364. Wildfeur A, Mayerhofer D. The effects of **plant** preparations on cellular functions in body defense. Arzneimittelforschung. 1994; 44(3):361-6. See also ref. 316.
365. Shekelle P, Adams A, et al. Spinal manipulation for **low back pain**. Ann Int. Med. 1997; 117(7):590-8.
366. Carey T, Garrett J, et al. The outcomes and costs of care for acute low **back pain** among patients seen by primary care practitioners, chiropractors, and orthopedic surgeons. NEJM 1995; 333:913-7.
367. Assendelft W, Bouter L, Knipschild P. **Complications** of spinal manipulations. J Fam Pract. 1996; 5:475-80.
368. Lee K, Carlini W, et al. Neurologic complications following **chiropractic** manipulation. Neurology 1995; 45(6):1213-5.
369. Boik, J. *Cancer & Natural Medicine.* Princeton, MN: Oregon Medical Press. 1995.
370. Gray N. Evidence and overview of global **tobacco** problem. J Natl Canc Inst Monogr. 1992; 12:15-16.
371. White C. Research on **smoking** and lung cancer: a landmark in the history of chronic disease epidemiology. Yale J Biol Med. 1990; 63(1):29-46.
372. Bartram T. *Encyclopedia of Herbal Medicine*, 1st ed. Christchurch, Dorset: Grace Publishers, 1995.
373. Hoffman D. An Elder's Herbal. Rochester, Vermont: Healing Arts

374. Brown D. ***Herbal Prescriptions for Better Health.*** Rocklin, CA: Prima Publishing, 1996.
375. Spiegel D. Psychosocial aspects of **breast cancer** treatment. Semin. Oncol. 1997: 24(1 Suppl 1):S1-S36, S147.
376. Goodwin P, Leszcz M, et al. Randomized trial of group psychosocial support in metastatic **breast cancer**: the BEST study. Breast-Expressive supportive therapy study. Cancer Treat Rev 1996; 22 (Suppl A): 91-6.
377. Grundmann E. **Cancer morbidity and mortality** in USA Mormons and Seventh-day Adventists. Arch Anat Cytol Pathol 1992; 40(2-3):73-8.
378. Fraser G. Determinants of **ischemic heart disease** in Seventh-day Adventists: a review. Am J Clin Nutr 1988; 48(3 Suppl):833-36.
379. Beilin L, Rouse I, et al. **Vegetarian diet** and blood pressure levels: incidental or causal association? Am J Clin Nutr 1988; 48(3 Suppl):806-10.
380. Snowdon D. **Animal product consumption** and mortality because of all causes combined, coronary heart disease, stroke, diabetes, and cancer in Seventh-day Adventists. Am J Clin Nutr. 1988; 48(3 Suppl): 739-48.
381. Kupin V, Polevaia E. Stimulation of the immunological reactivity of cancer patients by **eleutherococcus** extract. Vopr Onkol 1986; 32(7):21-6.
382. Creagan E. **Attitude and disposition**: do they make a difference in cancer survival? Mayo Clin Proc 1997; 72(2):160-4.
383. Levin J. How **religion** influences morbidity and health: reflections on natural history, salutogenesis and host resistance. Soc Sci Med 1996; 43(5):849-64.
384. Jeffers L. Anesthetic considerations for the new **antiobesity medications**. AANA J 65(2):104.
385. Nightingale S. From the FDA. JAMA 1997; 278(5):379.
386. Sukkari S. Weighing benefits and risks of drugs to treat **obesity**. Can Med Assoc J. 1997; 156(6):768-9.
387. Cohen S, Doyle W, et al. Social ties and susceptibility to the **common cold**. JAMA 1997; 277(24):1940-44.
388. Cohen S, Tyrrell D, et al. Smoking, alcohol consumption, and susceptibility to the common **cold**. Am J Public Health 1993; 83(9):1277-83.
389. Cohen S, Tyrrell D, Smith A. Negative life events, perceived **stress**, negative affect, and susceptibility to the common cold. Br J Nutr 1997; 77(1):59-72.
390. Hemila H. **Vitamin C** intake and susceptibility to the common cold. Br J Nutr 1997; 77(1):59-72.
391. Avorn J, Monane M, et al. Reduction of bacteriuria and pyuria after ingestion of **cranberry** juice. JAMA 1994; 271(10):751-4.
392. Desenclos J, Abiteboul D, et al. Focus on the role of ventilation and ultraviolet rays in preventing nosocomial transmission of **tuberculosis** in health care facilities. Rev Pneumol Clin 1995; 51(1):13-21.
393. Hudelson P. Gender differentials in **tuberculosis**: the role of socio-economic and cultural factors. Tuber Lung Dis 1996; 77(5):391-400.
394. Kost R. **Postherpetic neuralgia** – pathogenesis, treatment and prevention. NEJM 1996; 335(1):32-42.

395. Gauvin L, Spence J. **Physical activity** and psychological well-being: knowledge base, current issues, and caveats. Nutr Rev. 1996; 54(4 Pt 2):S53-65.
396. Chien P. Magnesium sulphate in the treatment of eclampsia and pre-eclampsia: an overview of the evidence from randomised trials. Br J Obst Gyn 1996; (103)11:1085-91.
397. Zhang J, Bernasko J, et al. Continuous labor support from **labor attendant** for primiparous women: a meta-analysis. Obstet Gynecol 1996; 88(4 Pt 2):739-44.
398. Cunningham F. *Williams Obstetrics, 19th ed*. Norwalk, CT: Appleton & Lange,m 1993.
399. McLellan A, Grossman D, et al. **Acupuncture** treatment for drug abuse: a technical review. J Subst Abuse Treat 1993; 10(6):569-76.
400. Wolf S, Barnhart H, et al. Reducing frailty and falls in older persons: an investigation of **Tai Chi** and computerized balance training. J Am Geriatr Soc 1996; 44(5):489-97.
401. Field T. **Massage** therapy for infants and children. J Dev Behav. Pediatr 1995; 16(2):105-11.
402. Sanbongi C, Suzuki N, Sakane T. Polyphenols in **chocolate**, which have antioxidant activity, modulate immune functions in humans in vitro. Cell Immunol 1997; 177(2):129-36.
403. Kondok, Hirano R, et al. Inhibition of LDL oxidation by **cocoa**. Lancet 1996; 348(9040):1514.
404. diTomaso E, Beltramo M, Piomelli D. Brain cannabinoids in **chocolate**. Nature 1996; 382(6593):677-78.
405. Chou T, Benowitx N. Caffeine and **coffee**: effects on health and cardiovascular disease. Comp Biochem Physiol C Pharmacol Toxicol Endocr 1994; 109(2):173-89.
406. Duke, James. *The Green Pharmacy*. Emmaus, Penn: Rodale Press, 1997.
407. Benson, Herbert. *Timeless Healing. The Power and Biology of Belief*. New York: Simon & Schuster, 1996.
408. Dossey, Larry. **Healing Words**. San Francisco: Harper Collins Publishers, 1994.
409. Benson, Herbert. The **Relaxation Response**. New York: Avon Books, 1975.
410. Thom E, Woolan T. A controlled clinical study of Kanjang mixture in the treatment of uncomplicated upper **respiratory tract infections**. Phytotherapy Research 1997; 11:207-10. (Reviewed in FACT: Focus on Alternative and Complementary Therapies 1997; 2(3):111-2.
411. Ernst E. **Acupuncture**/Acupressure for weight reduction? A systemic review. Wien Klin Wochenschr 1997; 109/2:60-62.
412. Ernst E, White A. Life-threatening adverse reactions after **acupuncture**? A systematic review. Pain 1997; 71:123-6.
413. Ernst E, DeSmet P.A.G.M. **Risks** associated with complementary therapies. In *Meyler's Side Effects of Drugs, 13th Edition*. M.N.G. Dukes, ed. 1996: Elsevier Science B.V.
414. Ernst E. The attitude against **immunisation** within some branches of complementary medicine. Eur J Pediatr 1997. 156:513-5.
415. Bursztyn M, Mekler J, Ben-Ishay D. The **siesta** and ambulatory blood pressure: is waking up the same in the morning and afternoon? J Hum Hypertens 1996. 10(5):287-92.

416. Pack AI, Pack AM, et al. Characteristics of **crashes attributed to the driver having fallen asleep.** Accid Anal Prev 1995. 27(6):769-75.
417. Kim D, Eastman A, et al. **Fish oil**, atherogenesis, and thrombogenesis. Ann N Y Acad Sci 1995; 748:474-80.
418. Endres S, De Caterina R, et al. n-3 polyunsaturated **fatty acids**: update 1995. Eur J Clin Invest. 1995; 25(9):629-38.
419. Sacks F, Stone P, et al. Controlled trial of **fish oil** for regression of human coronary atherosclerosis. HARP Research Group. J Am Coll Cardiol 1995; 25(7):1492-8.
420 Mc Grath L, Brennan G, et al. Effect of dietary **fish oil** supplementation on peroxidation of serum lipids in patients with non-insulin dependent diabetes mellitus. Atherosclerosis 1996; 121(2):275-83.
421. Cukier C, Waitzberg D. Biological activity of **fish oil**. Arq Gastroenterol 1996; 33(3):173-8.
422. Kalmijn S, Feskens E, et al. Polyunsaturated **fatty acids**, antioxidants, and cognitive function in very old men. Am J Epidemiol 1997; 145(1):33-41.
423. Temple NJ. **Dietary fats** and coronary artery disease. Biomed Pharmacother 1996; 50(6-7):261-8.
424. Weisburger J. **Dietary fat** and risk of chronic disease: mechanistic insights from experimental studies. J Am Diet Assoc 1997; 97(7 Suppl):S16-23).
425. Slattery M, Potter J, et al. Plant foods and **colon cancer**: an assessment of specific foods and their related nutrients (United States). Cancer Causes Control 1997; 8(4):575-90.
426. Potter JD. Nutrition and **colorectal cancer**. Cancer Causes Control 1996; 7(1):127-46.
427. Loeb H, Vandenplas Y, et al. Tannin-rich **carob** pod for the treatment of acute-onset diarrhea. J Pediatr Gastroenterol Nutr 1989; 8(4):480-5.
428. Tarka SM Jr. The toxicology of **cocoa** and methylxanthines: a review of the literature. Crit Rev Toxicol 1982; 9(4):275-312.
429. Stahl W, Sies H. **Lycopene**: a biologically important carotenoid for humans? Arch Biochem Biophys 1996; 336(1):1-9.
430. Giovannucci E, Ascherio A, et al. Intake of carotenoids and retinol in relation to risk of **prostate cancer**. J Natl Cancer Inst. 1995; 87(23):1767-76.
431. Lubin F, Ron E, et al. A case-control study of caffeine and **methylxanthines** in benign breast disease. JAMA 1985; 253(16):2388-92.
432. Heyden S, Muhlbaier LH. Prospective study of "fibrocystic breast disease" and **caffeine** consumption. Surgery 1984; 96(3):479-84.
433. Birch, Stephen and Hammerschlag, Richard. *Acupuncture efficacy: a summary of controlled clinical trials.* 1997.
434. Baltrusch HJ, Stangel W, Titze I. **Stress, cancer** and immunity. Acta Neurol (Napoli) 1991; 13(4): 315-27.
435. Somer, Elizabeth. *Food & Mood.* New York: Henry Holt and Company, 1995.
436. Manoukian A, et al. Rhabdomyolysis secondary to lovastatin therapy. Clin Chem 1990; 36(12): 2145-7.
437. Yoshikawa T, et al. The protection of **coenzyme Q 10** against carbon tetrachloride hepatotoxicity. Gastroent Jpn 1981; 16(3): 281-5.

438. Zheng, W. et al. **Well-done meat** intake and the risk of breast cancer. J. National Cancer Inst. 1998; 90(22): 1724-9.
439. Key TJ, et al. A case-control study of **diet and prostate cancer**. Br J Cancer 1997; 76(5): 678-87.
440. Sigounas G, et al. S-allylmercaptocysteine inhibits cell proliferation and reduces the viability of erythroleukemia, breast, and prostate cancer cell lines. Nutr Cancer 1997; 27(2): 186-91.
441. Faculty, Developing Virtue Secondary School. **Buddhism**: A Brief Introduction. Burlingame, CA: Buddhist Text Translation Society, 1996.
442. Venerable Weragoda Sarada Maha Thero. Treasury of Truth: The Illustrated Dhammapada (verses 109 and 221).
443. Naidoo T. Health and health care—a **Hindu** perspective. Med Law 1989; 7(6): 643-7.
444. Ramamurthi B. Mentality and behavior in **India**. Acta Neurochir (Wien) 1995; 132(4): 199-201.
445. Gatrad A. **Muslim customs** surrounding death, bereavement, postmortem examinations, and organ transplants. BMJ 1994; 309(6953): 521-3.
446. Malik G, et al. **Ramadan** fasting—effects on health and disease. J Assoc. Physicians India 1996; 44(5): 332-4.
447. Doyle T, et al. The association of drinking water source and **chlorination by-products** with cancer incidence among postmenopausal women in Iowa: a prospective cohort study. Am J Public Health 1997; 87(7): 1168-76.
448. Telles S, et al. **Yoga for rehabilitation**: an overview. Indian J Med Sci 1997; 51(4): 123-7.
449. Nespor K. Psychosomatics of back pain and the use of **yoga**. Int J Psychosom 1989; 36(1-4): 72-8.
450. Lewith G, and Watkins A. Unconventional therapies in **asthma**: an overview. Allergy 1996; 51(11): 761-9.
451. Manchanda S and Narang R. Yoga and **coronary artery disease**. Indian Heart J. 1998; 50(2): 227-8.
452. Nespor K. **Pain management and yoga**. Int J Psychosom 1991; 38(1-4): 76-81.
453. Flora K et al. **Milk Thistle** (Silybum marianum) for therapy of liver disease. Am J Gastroenterology 1998; 93:139-43.
454. Asser S and R Swan. Child fatalities from **religion-motivated medical neglect**. Pediatrics 1998; 101(4 Pt 1): 625-9.
455. The National Council Against Health Fraud. NCAHF Newsletter March/April 1998 (21:2).
456. The National Council Against Health Fraud. NCAHF Newsletter July/Aug 1998 (21:4).
457. Elihu, et al. **Chelation therapy** in cardiovascular disease: ethylenediaminetetraacetic acid, deferoxamine, and dexrazoxane. J Clin Pharmacol 1998; 38:101-105.
458. Linde, Klaus et al. Are the clinical effects of homeopathy placebo effects? A meta-analysis of placebo-controlled trials. Lancet 1997; 350:834-43.
459. Langman M. **Homeopathy** trials: reason for good ones but are they warranted? Lancet 1997; 350(9081): 825.
460. Associated Press, 8/31/98, as reviewed in The NCAHF Newsletter, Sept/Oct 1998 (21:5).

461. Wirth, Daniel P. The significance of **belief and expectancy** within the spiritual healing encounter. Soc Sci Med 1995; 41(2):249-60.
462. Wirth, Daniel P. Implementing **spiritual heali**ng in modern medical practice. Advances, The J of Mind-Body Health 1993; (9:4): 69-81.
463. Bensoussan A, et al. Treatment of irritable bowel syndrome with Chinese Herbal Medicine. JAMA 1998; 280:1585-9.
464. Weiser M, et al. **Homeopathic vs. conventional treatment of vertigo**: a randomized double-blind controlled clinical study. JAMA 1998; 280:1552f.
465. Garfinkel M, et al. Yoga-based intervention for carpal tunnel syndrome: A randomized trial. JAMA 1998; 280:1601-3.
466. Horowitz H. The effectiveness of community water fluoridation in the United States. J Public Health Dent 1996; 56(5):253-8.
467. Spencer A, et al. **Water fluoridation** in Australia. Community Dent Health 1996; 13(Suppl 2):27-37.
468. Fox G, et al. **Chromium** picolinate supplementation for diabetes mellitus. J Fam Pract 1998; 46(1):83-6.
469. Singh J, et al. Dietary **fat and colon cancer** . . . Cancer Res 1997; 57(2):253-8.
470. Thys-Jacobs S et al. **Calcium carbonate and the premenstrual syndrome**: effects on premenstrual and menstrual symptoms. Am J Obstet Gynecol 1998; 179(2):444-52.
471. Lan C, et al. 12-month **Tai Chi training** in the elderly: its effect on health fitness. Med Sci Sports exerc 1998; 30(3): 345-51.
472. Henderson N, et al. The roles of exercise and fall risk reduction in the prevention of osteoporosis. Endocrinol Metab Clin North am 1998; 27(2): 369-87.
473. Masley S. Tai Chi Chuan. Arch Phys Med Rehabil 1998; 79(11): 1483.
474. Jin P. Efficacy of Tai Chi, brisk walking, meditation, and reading in reducing mental and emotional stress. J Psychosom Res 1992; 36(4): 361-70.
475. Kirsteins A, et al. Evaluating the safety and potential use of a weight-bearing exercise, **Tai Chi Chuan**, for rheumatoid arthritis patients. Am J Phys Med Rehabil 1991; 70(3): 136-41.
476. Zhou D. Preventive **geriatrics**: an overview from traditional Chinese medicine. Am J Chin Med 1982; 10(1-4_:32-9.
477. Zhou M, et al. Observation of **qi-gong** treatment in 60 cases of pregnancy-induced hypertension. Chung His I Chieh Ho Tsa Chih 1989; 9(1):4-5, 16-18.
478. Hewson M. **Traditional healers in southern Africa**. Ann Intern Med 1998; 128(12 Pt 1): 1029-34.
479. Nelson K. **Osteopathic** medical considerations of reflex sympathetic dystrophy. J Am Osteopath Assoc. 1997; 97(5): 286-9.
480. Reitman C, S. Esses. Conservative options in the management of spinal disorders, Part II. Exercise, education and manual therapies. Am J Orthop 1995; 24(3): 241-50.
481. Sucher B. Palpatory diagnosis and manipulative management of **carpal tunnel** syndrome. J Am Osteopath Assoc 1994; 94(8): 647-63.
482. Rogers J and PL Witt. The controversy of **cranial bone motion**. J Orthop Sports Phys Ther 1997; 26(2): 95-103.

483. Degenhardt B and ML Kuchera. Update on **osteopathic** medical concepts and the lymphatic system. J Am Osteopath Assoc 1996; 96(2): 97-100.
484. Abraham I. **Prolotherapy** for chronic headache. Headache 1997; 37(4):256.
485. Isaksson H. Enthusiasts can not be entrusted with research on **homeopathy**. Lakartidningen 1998; 95(28-29): 3200-02. (article in Swedish).
486. Altman, Ellen and Peter Hernon, editors. *Research Misconduct: issues, implications, and strategies.* Greenwich, CT: Ablex, 1998.
487. Powell T, et al. **Ma Huang** strikes again: ephedrine nephrolithiasis. Am J Kidney Dis 1998; 32(1): 153-9.
488. Chiotakakou-Faliakou E, et al. Biofeedback provides long-term benefit for patients with intractable, slow and normal transit constipation. Gut 1998; 42(4): 517-21.
489. Papantonio C. Alternative medicine and **wound healing**. Ostomy Wound Manage 1998; 44(4): 44-6.
490. Sharquie K, et al. Treatment of cutaneous leishmaniasis by direct current electrtotherapy: the Baghdadin device. J Dermatol 1998; 25(4): 234-7.
491. Leung C, et al. **Karaoke** therapy in the rehabilitation of mental patiens. Singapore Med J 1998; 39(4): 166-8.
492. Liu W, et al. The herbal medicine sho-saiko-to inhibits the growth of malignant melanoma cells . . . In J Oncol 1998; 12(6): 1321-6.
493. Grootenhuis M, et al. Use of alternative treatment in pediatric oncology. Cancer Nurs 1998; 21(4): 282-8.
494. Bullough V and B Bullough. Should nurses practice **therapeutic touch** . . . J Prof Nurs 1998; 14(4): 254-7.
495. Rosted P. The use of **acupuncture in dentistry**: a review of the scientific validity of published papers. Oral Dis 1998; 4(2): 100-104.
496. De Leo, V et al. Treatment of neurovegetative **menopausal** symptoms with a phytotherapeutic agent. Minerva Ginecol 1998; 50(5): 207-11.
497. Bittinger M et al. "Alternative" therapy methods in functional disorders of the gastrointestinal system. Z. Gastroenterol 1998; 36(6): 519-24. (article in German).
498. Dixon M. Does **'healing'** benefit patient with chronic symptoms? A quasi-randomized trial in general practice. J R Soc Med. 1998; 91(4): 183-8.
499. Coss R, et al. Alternative care. Patient choices for adjunct therapies within a cancer center. Cancer Pract 1998; 6(3): 176-81.
500. Stralka S, et al. Treatment of **hand and wrist pain**. A randomized clinical trial of high voltage pulsed, direct current built into a wrist splint. AAOHN J 1998; 46(5): 233-6.
501. McCleane G. The successful use of spinal cord stimulation to alleviate intractable **angina** pectoris. Ulster Med J 1998; 67(1): 59-60.
502. Mir L, et al. Effective treatment of cutaneous and subcutaneous malignant tumors by electrochemotherapy. Br J Cancer. 1998; 77(12): 2336-42.
503. Ramirez L. Electrochemotherapy on **liver tumours** in rabbits. Br J Cancer 1998; 77(12): 2104-11.

504. Ivanov K, et al. The use of **transcutaneous electrostimulation in the treatment of diabetic angioneuropathy**. VoprKurortol Fizioter Lech Fiz Kult 1998; (2): 30-31.
505. Kuznetsov O, et al. The comparative effects of classic massage of different intensities on patients with chronic salpingo-oophoritis. Vopr Kurortol Fizioter Lech Fic Kult 1998; (2): 20-23.
506. Lal S, et al. Effect of feedback signal and psychological characteristics on **blood pressure** self-manipulation capability. Psychophysiology 1998; 35(4): 405-12.
507. Seidl M, et al. Alternative treatments for **menopausal symptoms**. Systematic review of scientific and lay literature. Can Fam Physician 1998; (44): 1299-1308.
508. Julka I. Beneficial effects of electrical stimulation on neuropathic symptoms in diabetic patients. J Foot Ankle Surg 1998; 37(3): 191-4.
509. Field T, et al. **Burn injuries** benefit from massage therapy. J Burn Care Rehabil 1998; 19(3): 241-4.
510. Greeff A, et al. Use of **progressive relaxation** training for chronic alcoholics with insomnia. Psychol Rep 1998; 82(2): 407-12.
511. Buckel P. Toward a new natural medicine. Naturwissenschaften 1998; 85(4): 155-63.
512. Henneberg A. Additional therapies in **Parkinson's disease** patients: useful tools for the improvement of the quality of life or senseless loss of resources? J Neurol 1998; 245(Suppl 1): s23-7.
513. Leigh E. **St. John's wort** (hypericum perforatum): the "depression herb" herb Research News 1997; (2:2), p. 4.
514. Kanowski S, et al. Proof of efficacy of the **Ginkgo biloba** special extract Egb761 in outpatients suffering from mild to moderate primary dementia of the Alzheimer type or multi-infarct dementia. Phytomedicine 1997; 4(1): 3-13.
515. Webb G. Indian Herb for chronic **congestive heart failure**. Herbal Gram 1997; (41): 21.
516. Maggioni M et al. Effects of **phosphatidylserine** therapy in geriatric patients with depressive disorders. Acta Psychiatr Scand 1990; 81(3): 265-70.
517. Crook T, et al. Effects of phosphatidylserine in age-associated **memory impairment**. Neurology 1991; 41(5): 644-9.
518. Cenacchi T, et al. Cognitive decline in the elderly: a double-blind, placebo-controlled multicenter study on efficacy of **phosphatidylserine** administration. Aging (Milano) 1993; 5(2): 123-33.
519. Khalsa DS. Integrated medicine and the prevention and reversal of memory loss. Altern Ther Health Med 1998; 4(6): 38-43.
520. Boesler D, et al. Efficacy of high-velocity low-amplitude manipulative technique in subjects with **low-back pain** during menstrual cramping. J Am Osteopath Assoc 1993; 93(2): 203-8, 213-4.
521. MacDonald RS and CM Bell. An open controlled assessment of osteopathic manipulation in nonspecific low-back pain. Spine. 1990; 15(5): 364-70.
522. Williams N. Managing **back pain** in general practice—is osteopathy the new paradigm? Br J Gen Pract 1997; 47(423): 653-5.
523. Allen T, et al. Investigating the role of **osteopathic manipulation** in the treatment of asthma. J Am Osteopath Assoc. 1993; 93(6): 654-6, 659.

524. Sucher B. Palpatory diagnosis and **manipulative management of carpal tunnel** syndrome. J Am Osteopath Assoc. 1994; 94(8): 647-63.
525. Gosman-Hedstrom G, et al. Effects of **acupuncture** treatment on daily life activities and quality of life: a controlled, prospective, and randomized study of acute stroke patients. Stroke 1998; 29(10): 2100-8.
526. Chen L, et al. The effect of location of transcutaneous electrical nerve stimulation on postoperative opioid analgesic requirement: acupoint versus nonacupoint stimulation. Anesth Analg 1998; 87(5): 1129-34.
527. Honjo H, et al. Acupuncture for urinary incontinence in patients with chronic spinal cord injury: a preliminary report. Nippon Hin Yokika Gakkai Zasshi 1998; 89(7): 665-9.
528. Tempfer C, et al. Influence of **acupuncture** on maternal serum levels of interleukin-8, prostaglandin F2 alpha, and beta-endorphin: a matched pair study. Obstet Gynecol 1998; 92(2): 245-8.
529. Guimaraes CM, et al. Effects of acupuncture on behavioral, cardiovascular and hormonal responses in restraint-stressed Wister rats. Braz J Med Biol Res 1997; 30(12): 1445-50.
530. Ternov K, et al. Acupuncture for pain relief during **childbirth**. Acupunct Electrother Res 1998; 23(1): 19-26.
531. Furugard S, et al. Acupuncture worth trying in severe **tinnitus**. Lakartidningen 1998; 95(17): 1922-8.
532. Abuaisha BB, et al. Acupuncture for the treatment of chronic painful peripheral diabetic neuropathy: a long-term study. Diabetes Res Clin Pract 1998; 39(2): 115-21.
533. Li P, et al. Reversal of reflex-induced **myocardial ischemia** by median nerve stimulation: a feline model of electroacupuncture. Circulation 1998; 97(12): 1186-94.
534. Sanchez-Araujo M, A. Puchi. **Acupuncture** enhances the efficacy of antibiotics treatment for canine otitis crises. Acupunct Electrother Res 1997; 22(3-4): 191-206.
535. Ernst E. Acupuncture as a symptomatic treatment of **osteoarthritis**. A systematic review. Scand J Rheumatol 1997; 26(6): 444-7.
536. Ernst E, et al. Complementary therapies for **depression**: an overview. Arch Gen Psychiatry 1998; 55(11): 1026-32.
537. Podmore I, et al. **Vitamin C** exhibits pro-oxidant properties. Nature 1998; 9:392 (6676): 559.
538. Powell T, et al. **Ma-huang** strikes again: ephedrine nephrolithiasis. Am J Kidney Dis 1998; 32(1): 153-9.
539. Herrera J, et al. Prevention of **preeclampsia** by linoleic acid and calcium supplementation: a randomized controlled trial. Obstet Gynec 1998; 91: 585-90.
540. Appel L, et al. A Clinical trial of the effects of dietary patterns on blood pressure. **DASH** Collaborative Research Group. NEJM 1997; 336(16): 117-24.
541. Bonnet M and D. Arand. We are chronically **sleep deprived**. Sleep 1995; 18(10): 908-11.
542. Hammond E. Some preliminary findings on physical complaints from **a prospective study of 1,064,004 men and women**. Am J Pub Health 1964; (54): 23.
543. Benca R and J Quintas. Sleep and host defenses: a review. Sleep 1997; 20(11): 1027-37.

544. Narkiewicz K, et al. The sympathetic nervous system and **obstructive sleep apnea**: implications for hypertension. J Hyperten 1997; 15(12-2_: 1613-9.
545. Lesske J et al. **Hypertension** caused by chronic intermittent hypoxia— influence of chemoreceptors and sympathetic nervous system. J Hyperten 1997; 15(12-2): 1593-1603.
546. Marcus C, et al. Blood pressure in children with **obstructive sleep apnea**. Am J Resp Crit Care Med 1998; 157(4-1): 1098-1103.
547. Edenharder R, et al. In vitro effect of **vegetable and fruit juices** on the mutagenicity of . . . Food Chem Toxicol 1994; 32(5): 443-59.
548. Rosa L et al. A Close look at **therapeutic touch**. JAMA 1998; 279: 1005-10.
549. Harvey M and M. Elliot. **Transcutaneous electrical nerve stimulation** for pain management during cavity preparations in pediatric patients. ASDC J Dent Child 1995; 62(1): 49-51.
550. Mellor A. A comparison of injectable local anesthesia and electronic dental anesthesia in restorative dentistry. Anesth Pain Control Dent 1993; 2(3): 177-9.
551. Roth N, et al. Psychophysiological assessment of transcutaneous electric nerve stimulation (**TENS**) effects upon orofacial pain. Biomed Biochim Acta 1990; 49(7): 613-8.
552. Stanko R, et al. Enhanced leg exercise endurance with a high-carbohydrate diet and **dihydroxyacetone and pyruvate**. J App Phys 1990; 69(5): 1651-6.
553. Vandebuerie F, et al. Effect of **creatine loading** on endurance capacity and sprint power in cyclists. Int J Sports Med 1998; 19(7): 490-5.
554. Krizkova L, et al. The effects of **flavonoids** on ofloxacin-induced mutagenicity in Euglena gracilis. Mutat Res 1998; 416(1-2): 85-92.
555. Sturmi J and D Diorio. **Anabolic agents**. Clin Sports Med 1998; 17(2): 261-82.
556. Rao M and V Sabbarao. Sex differences in **dehydroepiandrosterone**-induced hepatocarcinogenesis in the rat. Cancer Let 1998; 125(1-2):111-6.
557. Proctor D, et al. Age-related sarcopenia in humans is associated with reduced synthetic rates of specific muscle proteins. J Nutr 1998; 128(2 Suppl): 351S- 355S.
558. vanVollenhoven R, et al. Treatment os systemic lupus erythematosus with dehydroepiandrosterone: 50 patients treated up to 12 months. J Rheumatol 1998; 25(2): 285-9.
559. Han D, et al. **DHEA** treatment reduces fat accumulation and protects against insulin resistance in male rats. J Gerontol A Biol Sci Med Sci 1998; 53(1): B19-24.
560. Labrie F, et al. Effect of 12-month **dehydroepiandrosterone** replacement therapy on bone, vagina, and endometrium in postmenopausal women. J Clin Endocrinol Metab 1997; 82(10): 3498-3505.
561. Swierczynski J, et al. Dietary **alpha-tocopherol** prevents dehydroepiandrosterone-induced lipid peroxidation in rat liver microsomes and mitochondria. Toxicol Lett 1997; 91(2): 129-36.
562. Josefson, D. Concern raised about **performance enhancing drugs** in the US BMJ 1998; (317): 702.

563. Kohlmeier L. Biomarkers of **fatty acid exposure and breast cancer** risk. Am J Clin Nutr 1997; 66(6 Suppl): 1548S-1556S.
564. Ip C. Review of the effects of **trans fatty acids**, oleic acid, n-3 polyunsaturated fatty acids, and conjugated linoleic acid on mammary carcinogenesis in animals. Am J Clin Nutr 1997; 66(6 Suppl): 1523S-1529S.
565. Kohlmeier L, et al. Adipose tissue **trans fatty acids and breast cancer** in the European Community Multicenter Study on Antioxidants, Myocardial Infarction, and Breast Cancer. Cancer Epidemiol Biomarkers Prev 1997; 6(9): 705-10.
566. Bakker N, et al. Adipose **fatty acids and cancers** of the breast, prostate and colon: an ecological study. EURAMIC Study Group. Int J Cancer 1997; 72(4): 587-91.
567. Aikins M. Alternative therapies for **nausea and vomiting of pregnancy**. Obstet Gynecol 1998; 91(1): 149-55.
568. Taylor R. Antibacterial constituents of the Nepalese medicinal herb, **Centipeda minima**. Phytochemistry 1998; 47(4): 631-34.
569. Vallbona C. Response of pain to static **magnetic fields** in post polio patients: A double-blind pilot study. Arch Phys Med Rehabil 1997; 78:1200-3.
570 Lautermann J, et al. **Glutathione** protection against gentamycin ototoxicity depends on nutritional status. Hear Res 1995; 86(1-2): 15-24.
571. White E, et al. Screening of potential cancer preventing chemicals as **antioxidants** in an in vitro assay. Anticancer Res 1998; 18(2A): 769-73.
572. DeLorgeril M, et al. **Mediterranean dietary** pattern in a randomised trial: prolonged survival and possible reduced cancer rate. Arch Intern Med 1998; 158: 1181-7.
579. Bay F. **Anthroposophical medicine**: a nursing perspective. Complent Ther Nurs Midwifery 1997; 3(6): 152-3.
580. The **heart** is not a pump: a refutation of the pressure propulsion premise of heart function. Frontier Perspectives, Fall/Winter 1995; 5(1): 15-24.
581. Ryan. History of **Ayurveda**. Arlington, VA: TM-EX; c. 1990.
582. Vita A, et al. **Aging, health risks, and cumulative disability**. NEJM 1998; 338: 1035-41.
583. Van Dalen DB and BL Bennett. *A World History of Physical Education*. Prentice Hall, 1971, p. 89-90.
584. Dubos R. *Mirage of Health*. Harper & Row. 1959.
585. Garrison F. *The History of Medicine*. Saunders 1929.
586. National College of Naturopathic Medicine Catalog 1984-85.
587. EEOC Notice, N-915.022.
588. Brierton TD. Employer's **new age** training programs fail to alter the consciousness of the EEOC. Labor Law Journal, July, 1992: 411-20.
589. Cherkin, et al. A comparison of physical therapy, chiropractic manipulation, and provision of an educational booklet for the treatment of patients with **low back pain**. NEJM 1998; 339: 1021-9.
590. Balon et al. A comparison of active and simulated **chiropractic** manipulation as an adjunctive treatment for childhood asthma. NEJM 1998; 339-20.

591. McGraw D. A **pink Viagra**? US News & World Report, 10/5/98: 54. (As reviewed in the NCRHI Newsletter Nov/Dec 1998; 21:6. The National Council for Reliable Health Information).
592. Sampson W and W London. Analysis of **homeopathic treatment** of childhood diarrhea. Pediatrics 96(5): 961-4.
593. Leng G et al. Exercise for **intermittent claudication**. The Cochrane Library—1998 issue 1, p. 1-13.
594. Ernst E. Harmless **Herbs**? A review of the recent literature. Am J Med. 1998; 104:170-8.
595. Ernst E. The heresy of **homeopathy**. A brief history of 200 years of criticism. British Homeopathic Journal 1998; 87: 28-32.
596. Ernst E. **Cancer Diets**: Fads and Facts. Cancer Prevention International 1996; 2:181-7.
597. Ernst E. **Chelation therapy** for peripheral arterial occlusive disease: a systematic review. Circulation 1997; 96:1031-3.
598. Ernst E and M. Pittler. **Yohimbine** for erectile dysfunction: a systematic review and meta-analysis of randomized clinical trials. The J. of Urology 1998; 159: 433-6.
599. McCutcheon L. What's that I smell? The claims of **aromatherapy**. Skeptical Inquirer 1996: May/June: 35-37.
600. Godfroid I. Eulogy of wine? Presse Med 1997; 26(40): 1971-4.
601. Orgogozo J, et al. **Wine** consumption and dementia in the elderly . . . Rev Neurol (Paris) 1997; 153(3): 185-92.
602. Eisenberg D, et al. "**Unconventional" medicine** in the United States—**prevalence**, costs and patterns of use. NEJM 1993; 328:246-52.
603. Proverbs 3:3 (Bible)
604. Safran D, et al. Linking **primary care** performance to outcomes of care. J Fam Pract 1998; 47(3): 213-20.
605. Relman, Arnold S. **A Trip to Stonesville. Andrew Weil, the boom in alternative medicine, and the retreat from science.** The New Republic. Dec. 14, 1998.
606. Mackay, Charles. *Extraordinary Popular Delusions and the Madness of Crowds.*
607. Kleijnen J, et al. **Placebo** effect in double-blind clinical trials: a review of interactions with medications. Lancet 1994; 344: 1347-49.
608. Melchart D, Linde K, et al. The **integration of natural healing** procedures into research and teaching at German universities. Altern Ther Health med 1995; 1(1): 30-3.
609. Armitage P and G Berry. **Statistical Methods** in Medical Research, 3rd ed. (p. 194-5). Oxford: Blackwell Scientific Publications, 1994.
610. Paramore LC. **Use of Alternative Therapies**: Estimates from the 1994 Robert Wood Johnson Foundation National Access to Care Survey. J Pain Symptom Manage 1997; 13:83-9.
611. Andrews L, et al. The use of alternative therapies by **children with asthma**: a brief report. J Paediatr Child Health 1998; 34: 131-4.
612. Ter Riet G, et al. Is **placebo** analgesia mediated by endogenous opiods? A systematic review. Pain 1998; 76: 273-275.
613. Astin J. **Why patients use alternative** medicine: results of a national study. JAMA 1998; 279: 1548-53.

ABBREVIATIONS USED

ac: before meals
ADA: American Dietetic Association
adv.: adverse
AIDS: acquired immune deficiency syndrome
amt.: amount
ANF: atrial natriuretic factor
AODM: adult onset diabetes mellitus
ASA: aspirin
BID: twice a day
BP: blood pressure
BPH: benign prostatic hypertrophy
CA: cancer
CAD: coronary artery disease
cf.: compare with
CHF: congestive heart failure
CI: contra-indicated
CMV: cytomegalovirus
CNS: central nervous system
CTX: contractions
CV: cardiovascular
Δ: change
div.: divide (into)
Δ: change
DM: diabetes mellitus
dz: disease
etoh: ethanol
extr.: extract
FDA: U.S. Food and Drug Administration
g: gram
GERD: gastro-esophageal reflux disease
GI: gastrointestinal
GRAS: generally recognized as safe
 (by the FDA)
HA: headache
HDL: high density lipoprotein
HR: heart rate
HTN: hypertension
IBS: irritable bowel syndrome
IM: intra-muscular
incl: including
IV: intravenous
K: potassium
LD_{50}: lethal dose in 50% of cases
LDL: low density lipoprotein
LFT: liver function test
MAO-I: mono-amine oxidase inhibitor
mg: milligram

mod: moderate
MS: multiple sclerosis
M.S.: master's in science degree
muc. mem.: mucous membranes
NCAHF: National Council Against Health Fraud
N/V/D: nausea/vomiting/diarrhea
occl.: occasional
PFT: pulmonary function test
PMS: pre-menstrual syndrome
PO: per os (by mouth)
PRL: prolactin
PUD: peptic ulcer disease
pulm.: pulmonary
PVR: peripheral vascular resistance
QD (or qd): once a day
QID: four times a day
RCT: randomized controlled trial
rbc: red blood cell
R'x: prescription
Ref.: reference
Resp.: respiratory
sl: slight
SLE: systemic lupus erythematosis
temp: temperature
TID: three times a day
top: topical
trigl.: triglycerides
usu.: usually
UTI: urinary tract infection
vv: varicose veins
wbc: white blood cell (usu. Refers to count)
xs: excess
ψ: psychiatric

INDEX

abbreviations-163
acacia gum-81
acne- 59
acerola- 81
acidophilus-81
aconite-81
acupressure- 31, 72
acupuncture- 20-22
addictions- 21, 72
adolescent- 73
aging- 70
African religions- 76
agrimony- 81
alchemilla - 81
alcohol- 63
aletris- 81
alfalfa- 81
allergies- 63, 68
allopathy- 36
allspice- 81
aloe- 82
alpinia- 82
altruism- 35
Alzheimer's- 71
ammi- 57, 82
androstenedione - 48
anemia- 56, 63
angelica- see dong quai
anger- 52, 53, 77
angina- 56
anthroposophical med.-22
antioxidants- 47, 52, 63
anxiety- 56, 73
aphrodisiacs- 63, 67, 73
apple- 82
arnica- 82
aroma therapy- 23
arsenic- 112
art- 23
arthritis- 47, 74
artichoke- 83
asparagus- 83
aspidium- 83
asthma- 74
atherosclerosis- 57-58
athletic- 48-49, 63
attention deficit- 73
autumn crocus- 83
avocado- 57, 60

ayurveda- 23
back- 21, 31, 50, 51, 74
barberry - 83
barley- 57
bayberry- 83
bearberry- 83
bee pollen- 83
bee venom- 84
berberine- 61
bergamot- 84
beta-carotene- 46
betel nut- 84
betony- 84
bilberry fruit- 84
biofeedback- 34
bioflavonoids- 84
biotin- 112
black cohosh- 85
black haw- 67
blindness- 72
blood type diet- 43
bloodroot- 85
blue cohosh- 85
blueberry- 85
boldo- 85
boneset- 85
boron- 112
Boswellia—see Frankincense
brewer's yeast- 57, 85
bromine- 113
broom- 86
buchu- 86
Buddhism- 76
burdock- 86
butcher's broom- 86
cabbage- 61
cadmium- 113
cajeput- 86
calabar bean- 86
calamus- 86
calcium- 46, 113
calendula officinalis (pot marigold)-86

canaigre- 86
cancer-42, 47, 52ff
candidiasis- 67
capers- 86
capsicum pepper- 86
cardamom- 87

carnitine- 49
carob- 87
carpal tunnel- 50, 128
carrot - 57, 87
cascara- 57, 87
castor- 87
cat's claw- 87
caution- 19
celery- 87
Centipeda minima- 87
chamomile- 88
chaparral- 88
charcoal- 88
chaste tree- 88
chelation- 23
chestnut- 59, 98
chi- 20
chicory- 88
Chinese medicine- 20, 30, 88
chiropractic- 24
chloride- 114
chlorination- 52
chocolate- 89
cholesterol- 57
choline- 49
chromium- 48, 114
chronic fatigue- see fatigue
cinnamon- 89
clematis- 89
clove- 90
CNS- 71
cocoa- 89
coenzyme Q- 90
coffee- 90
cola- 90, 91
cold, common- 62
coltsfoot- 91
comfrey- 91
congestive heart failure- 58
constipation- 39, 60
copper- 115
cordyceps sinensis- 91
coriander- 91
coronary artery disease- 39, 47
coumadin- 45, 131, 132
counseling patients- 8
cramps (leg)- 64
cramps (menstrual)- 50, 67
cranberry- 91
creatine- 48

credentials- 9
critique of therapies- 20-51
cucumber, Chinese- 91
cumin- 92
CVA- 71, 72
damiana- 92
dandelion- 92
DASH diet-37
death, causes of- 30
death/dying-63, 77
decoction- 27
dehydration-61
dementia- 71
dental- 59
depression- 21, 73
dermatology- 59-60
devil's claw - 92
devil's club- 92
devil's dung- 92
DHEA- 49
diabetes mellitus-21, 39, 62, 71
diarrhea- 61
diet- 37-45, 64, 65
digestive system- 60-62
digitalis- 92
dihydroxyacetone— 49
disclaimer- 19
dolomite- 92
dong quai- 92
dualism- 33-34
dysmenorrhea- 67
ear, nose and
 throat- 62
echinacea- 93
elderberry- 93
elderly- see longevity
electromagnetic radiation- 24
eleutherococcus- 93
empathy- 23
endocrine system- 62
endorphins- 14, 20
enemas- 23
ephedra- 93
epilepsy- 71
essential fatty acids- 115, 118, 119
evening primrose- 57, 94
exercise- 25-26, 48-49, 57
faith- 75
fatigue- 63
Feingold diet- 73
fennel- 94
fenugreek - 57, 94

Index

fever- 64
feverfew- 94
fibromyalgia- 21, 74
fish oil- 46, 47
flax- 57, 94
fluoride- 47, 115
fluoridation - 47
folic acid (folate; folacin)- 45, 116
fo-ti- 94
frankincense- 95
fumitory- 95
galangal (alpinia)- 95
ganoderma (reishi)- 95
garlic- 57, 95
gelsemium- 96
General
 considerations- 20
genito-urinary system- 67
gentian- 96
GERD- 39, 61
germanium- 116
ginger- 96
ginkgo biloba- 96
ginseng- 57, 96
glucomannan- 57, 96
glucosamine- 97
goldenseal- 97
gotu kola- 97
grape seed- 97
green tea- 97
grief- 23
grifola- 100
guar gum- 98
guarana- 98
guggul- 57, 98
gymnema- 98
gynecology- 67
habits- 29, 30, 70
hawthorn- 98
heart disease - 56-58
helping others- 35
hepatitis- 61
herbs (see also name of herb)- 26, 27, 81-111
herpes- 69
hibiscus- 98
Hinduism- 78
HIV- 69
homeopathy- 27-29
honey- 98
horehound- 98

horse chestnut- 98
horsetail- 98
humor - 34
hypericum- see St. John's wort
hyperlipidemia- 39, 57
hypertension- 37, 58
hypnotherapy- 35
hyssop- 99
immune system - 34, 68
immunity- 68
infectious disease-68ff
infertility- 67
infusion- 27
insect repellent- 64
insomnia- 50, 64, 71
introduction- 12
iodine- 116
iron- 42, 117
irradiation of food- 48
irritable bowel- 38, 61
Islam - 78
jet lag- 64
jewelweed- 99
Jews; Jewish faith - 30, 78
jojoba- 99
juniper- 99
karaya gum- 99
kava-kava- 99
ketogenic diet- 71
key- 18
khat- 99
kidney (nephropathy) - 47, 56
kudzu- 99
laminaria (kelp)- 100
lavender - 100
lead- 117
leg cramps - 64
lemon verbena- 100
lemongrass- 100
lentinan - 69
lice- 70
licorice- 100
lifestyle- 29, 52, 62
light therapy- 25
linden- 100
linoleic acid- 118
linolenic acid- 119
lithium- 119
longevity- 70
lovage- 100
love- 78
lupus- 74

Index

mace- 100
magnesium- 120
magnets - 24
maitake (grifola)- 57, 100
manganese- 121
marigold- see calendula
marijuana- 101
martial arts- 31
massage therapy - 31, 32
mate'- 101
medical-legal - 10
meditation- 35
Mediterranean diet- 42
melaleuca- 101
melatonin- 101
menopause- 67
milk thistle- 101
mind-body- 32
mistletoe- 101
molybdenum- 121
monascus - 57, 101
Mormon - 30
moxibustion- 20
mullein- 102
multiple sclerosis- 71
mushrooms- 53
music - 35
musk- 56
myocardial infarction - 58
myricetin- 102
myrrh- 102
National Council For Reliable
    Health Information - 20, 133
natural hygiene - 35
naturopathy- 36-37
nausea- 56
neem- 102
neonatal- 31
neopaganism - 51
nervous system- 71
New Age - 51
nickel- 121
nocebo- 20
noni
(morinda citrifolia)- 102
nutmeg- 102
nutrients (see also nutrition)- 112-132
nutrition- 37-49, 112-132
nuts- 58
oats- 57, 102
obesity - 39, 64-66
obstetrics- 72

occupational medicine- 66
octacosanol- 102
olive- 42
ophthalmology- 72
Optimum Health Diet Plan - 38-41
ordering
information- **www.boitumelo.com**
oregano- 103
Ornish (diet)- 42
orthopedics- 74, 79
osteopathic med.- 49
osteoporosis- 26, 71
pain- 21, 66
Pao d' Arco- 103
parsley- 61
passion flower- 103
patient education- 134
pectin- 57, 103
pediatrics- 31-32, 35
pennyroyal- 103
pepper (black)- see capsicum
peppermint - 103
peptic ulcer- 61
perilla- 57
peripheral vascular disease-58
peru balsam- 103
peyote- 103
phosphorous- 122
Phosphatidyl-serine— 71
pineapple- 62, 68
placebo - 14
plantain (psyllium)- 57
pomegranate- 67
potassium- 122
prayer- 75
pregnancy (see also obstetrics)- 45, 72
Premenstrual
syndrome- 46
primrose, evening-
see evening
primrose
prolotherapy - 50
Propolis- 104
psoriasis- 60
psychiatric- 72
psychology- 72
PTSD- 73
pumpkin seeds- 104
pycnogenol- 59, 74
pyrethrum- 104
pyruvate- 49
quantum theory - 14

quercetin-see bioflavonoids
quillaia- 104
quinine- 105
radiation- 24, 48, 66
raspberry- 61, 67
Raynaud's dz- 58
references- 135
reflexology- 31
rehabilitation- 72
reishi- 105
relaxation- 35
religion - 30, 34, 75-78
research methods - 12-16
respiratory system- 74
rest- 50, 64
Restless leg syn- 117
rheumatology- 74
rose hips- 105
rosemary- 105
royal jelly- 105
rubidium- 122
rue- 105
safflower- 57, 105
saffron- 105
sage- 105
sandalwood- 106
sassafras- 106
savory- 106
saw palmetto- 106
Scientific Quality Management - 13
schisandra- 106
schizophrenia- 73
scullcap- 106
seasonal affective disorder- 25, 73
sedentary - 30
seizures- 71
selenium- 46, 123
senna- 106
Seventh-day Adventist - 30
shark cartilage- 106
shiitake mushroom- 57, 106
siesta- 30
silicon- 123
silymarin- 107
skin cancer- 55
slippery elm- 107
smoking- 20, 29-30
soapwort- 107
social support- 53
sodium- 124
soy- 107
spirituality- 32-35, 53, 75
spirulina- 107

squill- 106, 107
St. John's Wort- 107
stinging nettle - 107
storax (styrax)- 108
strawberry- 67
stress- 66, 73
stroke (see CVA)
Sugar Busters™- 44
sulfur- 124
supplements - 45
surgery- 79
systems approach - 52
table of contents - 7
taheebo- 108
tai chi- 73
tansy- 108
tea tree- see melaleuca
therapeutic touch- 50-51
tin- 124
tincture- 27
tobacco- 30
tolu balsam- 108
tomato- 108
tonka bean - 108
toxins - 66
tragacanth- 108
trans fatty acids- 48
trauma- 79
travel information - 133
trillium- 108
tuberculosis- 70
turmeric- 109
turpentine (pine oil)- 109
unicorn root- see aletris
upside -down - 13
urinary tract infection- 67, 80
urology- 79-80
uva ursi- 109
vaginitis- 67
valerian- 109
vanadium- 125
vanilla- 109
varicose veins- 59
vegans- 42
vegetarian- 42, 76
vertigo- 66
Vitamin A- 125
Vitamin B1 (thiamine)- 125
Vitamin B2 (riboflavin)- 126

Index

Vitamin B3 (niacin)- 126
Vitamin B5 (pantothenic acid)-127
Vitamin B6 (pyridoxine)- 128
Vitamin B12 (cyanocobalamin)-42, 129
Vitamin C (ascorbic acid)- 130
Vitamin D- 131
Vitamin E (tocopherol)- 45, 46, 131
Vitamin K- 132
vitex- 88 (listed under chaste tree)
vomiting- 20, 56, 72
web sites- 133
weight table - 66
wellness- 64, 73
white cohosh- 109
wholism - 33-34
wine- 57, 110
wintergreen- 110
witch hazel- 110
withania- 110
woodruff-110
wormwood- 110
xylitol-62, 68
yam, wild- 110
yarrow- 110
yeast- see brewer's yeast
yellow dock- 111
yellow root-111
yerba santa- 111
yew- 111
yoga- 51
yogurt- 57
yohimbe- 111
yucca- 111
zinc- 42, 45, 49, 132
zone diet- 43